Intravascular ultrasound

Intravascular ultrasound

Techniques, developments, clinical perspectives

edited by

N. Bom
J. Roelandt

Rotterdam Postgraduate School of Cardiology

Kluwer Academic Publishers
Dordrecht / Boston / London

The articles in this publication have been reprinted from the
International Journal of Cardiac Imaging, Volume 4, Nos. 2–4, 1989 with
the original pagination of the journal.

ISBN-13: 978-94-010-6943-4   e-ISBN-13: 978-94-009-1007-2
DOI: 10.1007/978-94-009-1007-2

Printed on acid-free paper

Published by Kluwer Academic Publishers,
P.O. Box 17, 3300 AA Dordrecht, The Netherlands.

Kluwer Academic Publishers incorporates
the publishing programmes of
D. Reidel, Martinus Nijhoff, Dr W. Junk and MTP Press.

Sold and distributed in the U.S.A. and Canada
by Kluwer Academic Publishers,
101 Philip Drive, Norwell, MA 02061, U.S.A.

In all other countries, sold and distributed
by Kluwer Academic Publishers Group,
P.O. Box 322, 3300 AH Dordrecht, The Netherlands.

Editorial

New interventional techniques in vascular therapy include balloon dilatation, atherectomy and, for instance, laser ablation. The open arterial lumen can be studied angiographically. With this technique, however, little information on the obstruction itself becomes available. The new intervention methods have created a strong demand for techniques to visualize better the obstruction and the possible effect of therapy. Intravascular ultrasound has great potential to fill in this diagnostic demand.

Top experts in the field of intravascular ultrasound have jointly put together this publication which is the first to contain all the presently known aspects of this new, exciting field. The various chapters cover the full spectrum, which ranges from atherogenesis in arteries, through clinical applications, to aspects of more technical nature such as artifacts and catheter design. Although emphasis has been put on catheter tip imaging, intravascular Doppler blood velocity measurement techniques have also been included.

The main scope of this publication is to convey to the reader new ideas and possible clinical applications resulting from experience with today's fascinating new miniature catheter tip ultrasound imaging devices.

Rotterdam, June 1989

N. Bom, Ph.D.

Head Bioengineering
Thoraxcentre, Rotterdam and
Deputy Director of the
Interuniversity Cardiology
Institute of the Netherlands

J. Roelandt, M.D.

Head Dept. of Cardiology
Thoraxcentre, University
Hospital Rotterdam-Dijkzigt and
Erasmus University Rotterdam,
the Netherlands

Intravascular ultrasound is an exciting new area. Top experts have been asked to dedicate their efforts to compile together this first thorough book on catheter tip echography. Presentation of this book took place on the occasion of the 8th Symposium on Echocardiology held in Rotterdam, June 1989. The conference was organized in association with:

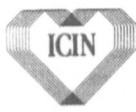 – the Interuniversity Cardiology Institute of the Netherlands

 – the Netherlands Heart Foundation

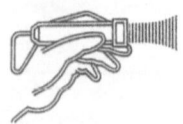 – the Dutch Society of Ultrasound in Medicine and Biology

Table of contents

VIII

International Journal of Cardiac Imaging **4**: 79–88, 1989.
© 1989 *Kluwer Academic Publishers.*

Early and recent intraluminal ultrasound devices

N. Bom[1,2], H. ten Hoff[1], C.T. Lancée[1], W.J. Gussenhoven[2] & J.G. Bosch[1]
[1] *Thoraxcentre, Erasmus University Rotterdam and* [2] *Interuniversity Cardiology Institute of the Netherlands,*
P.O. Box 1738, 3000 DR Rotterdam, the Netherlands

Abstract

The history of intraluminal echography dates back to the very beginning of diagnostic ultrasound. Over the years many fascinating ideas and applications of catheter tip or gastroscopic tube tip mounted transducers have been described. This chapter surveys these methods, subdividing them into a) measurements; b) Doppler and c) imaging. The survey ranges from early work of Cieszynski on the feasibility of echocardiography to more recent intra-arterial catheter tip Doppler with guidewire and balloon as described by Serruys.

Examples of ultrasound catheter tip echography in combination with other techniques such as angioscopy, laser ablation and spark erosion are also described. Today practical approaches are limited to imaging only. The three major approaches for catheter tip echo imaging are described and compared. This paper concludes with the results of automatic contour analysis of the inner arterial boundaries.

Introduction

Interventional catheter-based therapeutic techniques have recently become important as they may avoid the necessity of some surgical procedures. Techniques to widen a luminal obstruction in an artery include balloon dilatation, tip abrasion, atherectomy and laser ablation. The possibility that stenosis may reoccur is well documented. Apparently the therapeutic methods are not yet optimal, or cannot be optimally applied without further knowledge of the obstruction.

The arterial obstruction may consist of a variety of components, and geometric configurations. With contrast X-ray angiography only the remaining lumen can be visualized; not the obstruction itself.

A new and enthusiastic interest for intraluminal echography has been created in order to provide better patient selection and 'steering' of the interventional procedure. In addition, multi-purpose catheter tips, where echo is combined with a desobstruction method, have been suggested. For this purpose cross-sectional information is essential.

Angioscopy only allows visualizing of the innermost arterial layers. On the other hand, diagnostic ultrasound is well-known for cross-sectional imaging of soft tissue. Therefore, ultrasound seems like an ideal approach to image soft tissue such as the arterial wall or fibrotic plaque.

The strong interest in catheter tip echography has appeared only very recently. Nevertheless reports of intraluminal diagnostic ultrasound methods date back to the early fifties. Also in those days researchers described echographic methods where the acoustic element was mounted either on a catheter tip, gastroscopic pipe or other means for intraluminal diagnostic application of ultrasound.

In the early period of diagnostic ultrasound, one of the compelling reasons for the intraluminal approach was the low sensitivity of the existing echo transducers and, therefore the need to closely approach the organs to be studied.

A number of parameters exists which further favor the intraluminal approach. With higher frequency the wavelength becomes shorter. As a result the acoustic element can be small, still yielding a sufficient acoustic aperture in wavelength and thus acceptable beam characteristics. Due to the close approach to the reflecting structure, the increase in attenuation with frequency does not create a problem. The overall effect of the intraluminal approach is improvement of image resolution.

Early intraluminal measurements

The first applications of intraluminal echography were limited to the use of ultrasound for the purpose of echo travel-time measurement. In most of these applications, the focus was on organ dimensions or distances. No cross-sectional imaging or Doppler blood velocity imaging was reported. Early investigators and their approaches are schematically illustrated in Figs. 1 and 2.

In 1956, Cieszynski [1] built an ultrasonic catheter for intracardial investigation, and he was able to obtain ultrasonic reflections of soft tissues during model-experiments. In Fig. 1, the black area indicates the transducer element which has been mounted so that the sound beam is perpendicular to the catheter long axis.

In further experiments on dogs, he obtained good ultrasound reflections from the inner walls of the right and left ventricle as well as of the pulmonary artery. He noted that his method was harmless to the animals' health. This investigator concluded that new possibilities for the diagnosis of heart-failure in man might become possible with this method. Ten years later, Kossoff [2] described a catheter tip transducer of 2 mm diameter and operating frequency of 8 MHz for measuring intracardiac septal and ventricular wall thickness with an accuracy of up to 0.1 mm. He mentioned the movement of the catheter in the cardiac chamber as one of the problems. Peronneau [3] concluded in 1968 that the cavity to be measured does not generally have the form of a 'surface of resolution', and that two opposite acoustic elements instead of one should be mounted at the tip of a catheter. Thus by adding the thickness of the catheter to the sum of the two measurements the width of the cavity is obtained. Carleton [4] applied a 2.5 MHz cylindrical element of 3.1 mm outer diameter and radiating through a 360 degree arc. He distinguished two echoes, from the shortest and longest element-to-cardiac-chamber-wall-distance from which he derived chamber diameter in experiments on dogs. He also suggested adding a forward looking echo element.

In 1969, Stegall [5] introduced two transducers (0.7 × 1.5 mm) mounted at the end of a catheter-carried 'feeler gage' to determine intra-aortic and intracarotid diameter. It was a transit time system operating around 5 MHz. Another technique involved ultrasonic transit time measurement between two elements mounted at distance on a catheter. This technique was described by Kardon [6]. The catheter had to be manipulated so that it came to rest in a certain loop inside the ventricle. In 1974, Olson [7] described an esophageal device to monitor diameter and blood velocity at the same point

INTRALUMINAL MEASUREMENTS

Cieszynski	1956	single element echo	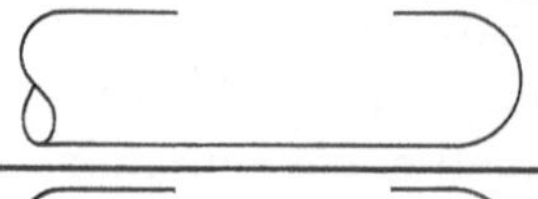	feasibility heart
Kossoff	1966	single element echo	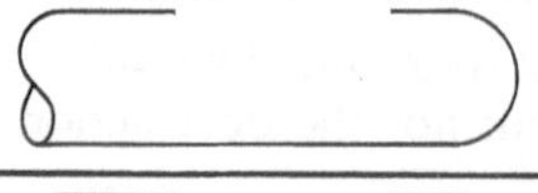	LV size septal thickness
Peronneau	1968	two elements	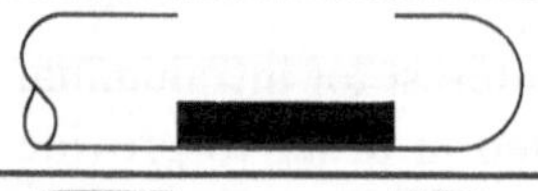	body cavity diameter
Carleton	1968	non-directional cylindrical element	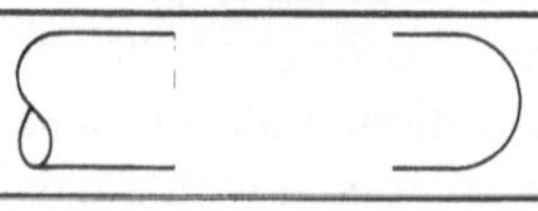	LV diameter

Fig. 1.

INTRALUMINAL MEASUREMENTS

Stegall	1969	transit time	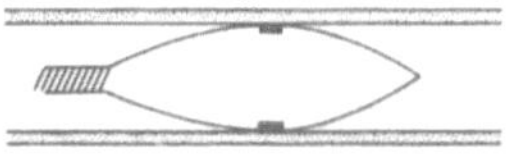	carotid diameter
Kardon	1971	transit time		LV diameter
Olson	1974	Doppler and echo	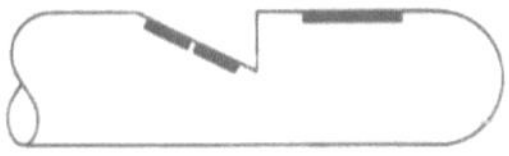	esophageal probe
Frazin	1976	M-mode registration	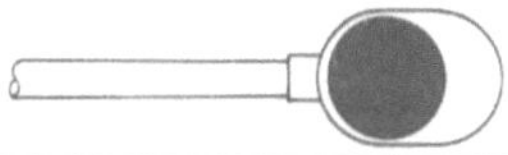	esophageal probe
Hughes	1978	3 elements	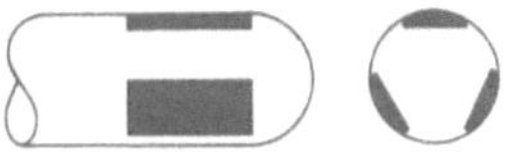	aortic lumen

Fig. 2.

along the ascending thoracic aorta. The probe was passed 1 to 2 cm distal to the aortic arch. Transesophageal cardiac M-mode registrations were described by Frazin [8]. He used a 9 mm 3.5 MHz transducer and studied cardiac structures in 38 subjects. In 1978, Hughes [9] increased the number of transducers from two to three to dynamically measure at 10 MHz the aortic lumen diameter.

Intravascular Doppler methods

It was well-known that frequency shift in reflected ultrasound waves may be used to measure blood velocity. With two transducer elements, one for transmission and one for reception, the so-called continuous wave Doppler technique was introduced. Blood velocity can be determined, but with continuous wave Doppler the sample depth at which the velocity is measured is ambiguous. With pulsed Doppler, introduced in the seventies, the measurement location could be identified as well. Presently, the combination of imaging with color Doppler has made precordial echo Doppler a clinically significant technique. A number of approaches have been described where Doppler methods were carried out through catheter mounting of the transducers.

Stegall described in 1967 [10] a continuous wave Doppler catheter which was used for instantaneous phasic coronary blood velocity measurement. A pulsed Doppler catheter tip version was introduced by Reid in 1974 [11]. The echo part could be inserted down the center of a 7 French catheter. Measurements were made in coronary and femoral arteries in dogs. Smaller sizes such as 5 French and high frequency (20 MHz) were introduced by Hartley [12] in 1974. He suggested an annular element. This set the way for Sibley [13] to combine this with a guide wire 12 years later.

Although mechanical rotation for imaging was introduced earlier, Gichard [14] first described a catheter construction with a rotating echo element mounted on a rotating flexible shaft in 1975 for Doppler purposes. The diameter of the probe was 3 mm. From here the step toward mechanically rotating catheter tip imaging devices seemed rather obvious.

Further concepts included work by Martin [15] to combine a forward looking Doppler (at 15 MHz) with transverse vessel area measurement in order to calculate blood flow. He describes an echo tip assembly with the possibility to use an inflatable balloon.

INTRAVASCULAR DOPPLER

Stegall	1967	continuous wave	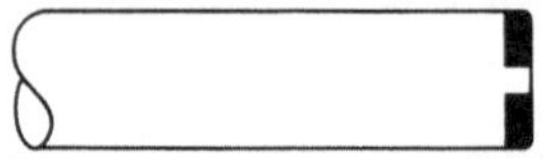	8 MHz	Fr 7-8
Reid	1974	pulsed	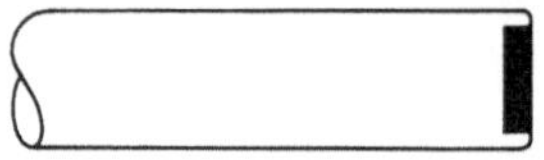	Fr 7	
Hartley	1974	pulsed annular element		20 MHz	Fr 5
Gichard	1975	rotating tip	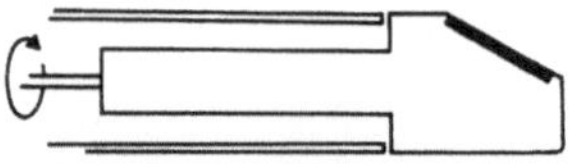	20 MHz	
Martin	1975	vessel area and Doppler	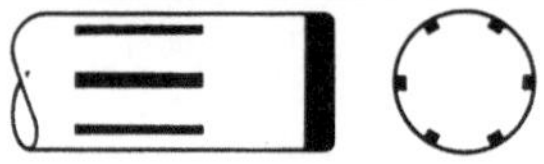	15 MHz	Fr 7
Sibley	1986	with guidewire	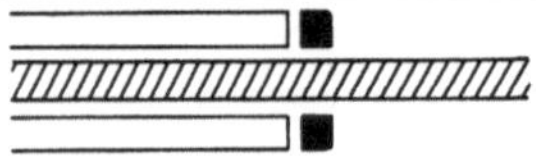	20 MHz	Fr 3-4

Fig. 3.

Intraluminal imaging

Already very early in the history of diagnostic ultrasound, information was used to form a cross-sectional image. For this purpose the acoustic beam had to scan through the cross-sectional plane. In order to obtain a realistic display the acoustic beam direction and beam deflection on the display had to be synchronized. Mechanically rotated transducers were used such as the one described by Wild [16] in 1955 for rectal tumor location.

Omoto [17] used an intravenous probe with guide wire tip to study cardiac structures, and Ebi-

INTRALUMINAL IMAGING

Wild	1955	echo-endoscope	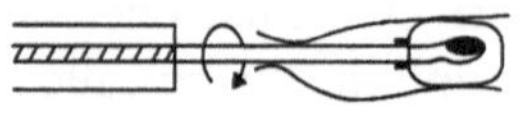	rectal tumour location
Omoto	1962	rotating probe C-scan	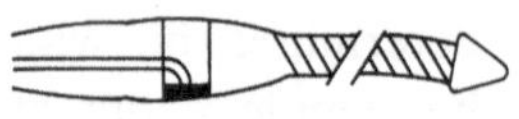	intracardiac tomography
Ebina	1964	transesophageal P.P.I. scanning	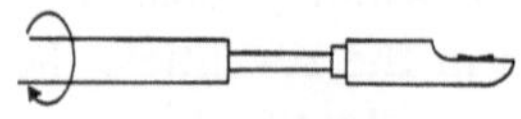	heart and vessels
Eggleton	1969	4-elements e.c.g. triggered	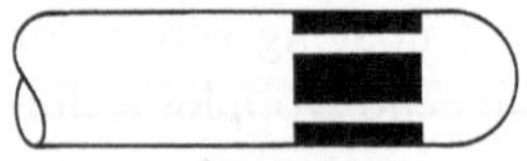	heart
Bom	1971	32-elements cylindrical phased array	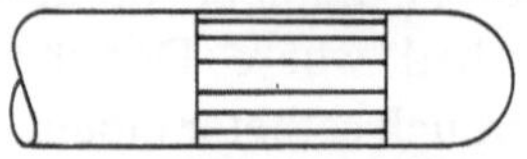	intracardiac tomography

Fig. 4.

na [18] described a miniature concave transducer for rotation inside a rubber cuff in the esophagus in 1964. Eggleton [19] approximated a cardiac cross section by rotating a 4-element catheter. Results of his system depended on a stable state of the heart since he accumulated data over many beats for reconstruction of a cross section in a selected steady state. As early as 1969 Bom [20] initiated a program to develop two-dimensional real-time invasive ultrasonic imaging using state-of-the-art technology. A 32-element circular phased array with an outer diameter of 3.2 mm mounted at the tip of a No. 9 French catheter (Fig. 5) was constructed. As pointed out in the original paper, the array design was a compromise between the optimal design and the limitations imposed by technological constraints. The final design was chosen to operate at 5.6 MHz with a narrow main beam. With this catheter real-time intraluminal images such as left ventricular cross-sections were recorded in the early seventies.

Today transesophageal echography has become of major importance in cardiology. Image quality is greatly improved if the attenuating chest structures can be avoided. Most of these systems have gastroscopic pipe mounted transducers. Some of the experience obtained with these systems has been used in development of smaller intraluminal devices. For example, Hisanaga [21] rotates a small trans-

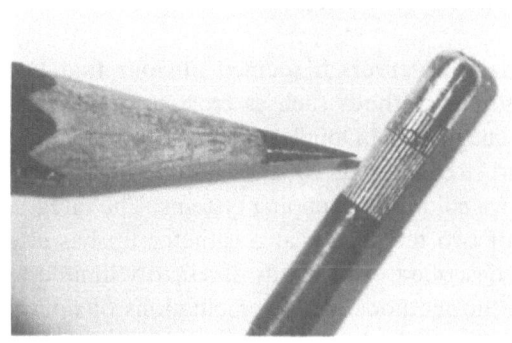

Fig. 5. The phased array 32-element catheter tip as described by Bom in the early seventies.

ducer fixed to a flexible shaft. It rotates at a rate of 15 to 50 cycles/s. DiMagno [22] adapts a 64-element linear array at 10 MHz. The field of view is 3 × 4 cm. Both Hisanaga and Bertini [23] use a distensible fluid filled bag for contact with the esophageal wall. Souquet introduced the phased array principle for esophageal applications in 1982 [24]. He even suggested forming an image in two perpendicular planes. Further applications of intraluminal imaging were described by Natori [25] and Fukuda [26] who were interested in the diagnosis of intra-abdominal disorders.

INTRALUMINAL IMAGING

Hisanaga	1977	transesophageal rotating scanner	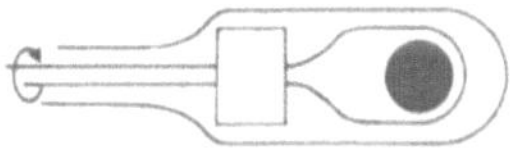	cardiac cross-sectional images
DiMagno	1980	64-elements	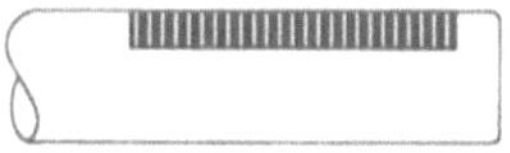	upper abdominal organs
Bertini	1981	distensible tip rotating catheter	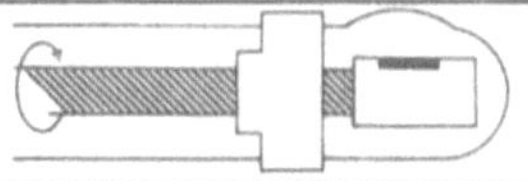	transesophageal cardiac
Souquet	1982	transesophageal phased array two-plane	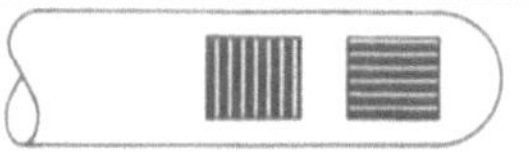	cardiac cross-sectional images
Natori	1982	transesophageal 5MHz linear array	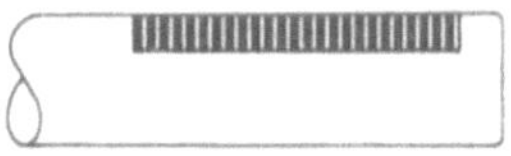	mediastinum

Fig. 6.

Combination of techniques

To many observers it seemed obvious that two ultrasound methods such as cross-sectional real-time imaging and Doppler blood velocity imaging should be combined. Today we see this in the non-invasive color flow mapping systems. The integration of two techniques at a catheter tip has also been described. This is not necessarily limited to two echo methods. Also combinations of optical inspection and ultrasound have been proposed. Given the pressing need to guide or monitor any intra-arterial obstruction removal technique, it seemed apparent that suggestions for the combination of removal techniques with ultrasound would appear. In the following a limited number of examples mainly obtained from patent applications, are presented in order to develop the present line of thinking in the existing field of intravascular echo imaging.

In the 'state-of-the-art' survey quoted by Nakada in 1983 [27] one of the many systems where cross-sectional echo is combined with optical inspection is shown in Fig. 7. The transducer (1) and the beam deflecting mirror (3) produce the cross-sectional image. The light source and reflections pass through optical fibers (2).

A combination of forward looking echo elements with laser ablation through a central fiber (1) is described by Webster [28] and shown in Fig. 8.

The positioning of the echo-elements (2) does not allow for imaging. It might yield six individual echo patterns with, no doubt, a difficult interpretation problem.

One possibility of combining echo with atherectomy is suggested by Yock [29] and shown in Fig. 9. A mechanically rotating transducer (1) and a rotating cutting element (2) are incorporated in a catheter with added guiding tip. An inflatable balloon can be used to press the atherectomy cutter towards the arterial obstruction.

Slager [30] described a recanalization method based on spark erosion. This can be used in a selective way to evaporate atherosclerotic plaque and other obstructions. It works well on fatty and fibrous tissue but still is in the experimental stage. Slager suggested a number of combinations with

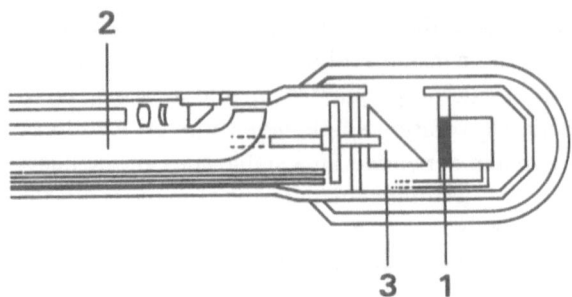

Fig. 7. Principle of echo catheter with optical viewing capability. The transducer (1); the fiber area (2) and the rotating mirror (3).

echo. One such example is shown in Fig. 10. The transducer (1) and the rotating beam-deflecting mirror (2) create the cross-sectional image. On the opposite side of the rotating tip a spark electrode can be positioned. Thus spark electrode and visualized obstruction are almost in the same plane. Other combinations of devices include the echo Doppler tip with a PTCA balloon catheter as described by Serruys [31]. After recording of the baseline intracoronary blood velocity in the proximal segment, the balloon catheter with Doppler probe at the tip was advanced over the stenosis and 3 to 7 inflations were applied to dilate the stenosis. Resting velocities before and after inflation were measured.

Present intra-arterial echo methods

The development of a miniature echo catheter whether based on a mechanically or electronically switched echo method presents severe technical problems. As a result all the suggested ideas for combining more than a single technique have not

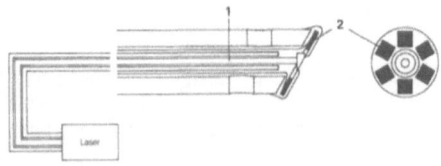

Fig. 8. A suggested combination of forward looking echo elements (2) with laser ablation through a fiber (1) (Webster; ref. [28]).

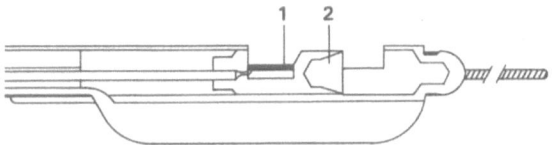

Fig. 9. Echographically guided atherectomy as proposed by Yock [29]. Element (1) and cutting mechanism (2).

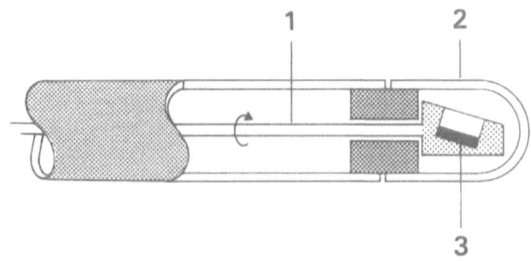

Fig. 11. Rotating shaft (1); transparent dome (2) and echo element (3) in a catheter tip system.

yet resulted in actual working models. Today researchers have put most of their effort into the diagnostic echo catheter tip alone. With these systems the first *in-vitro* and *in-vivo* results are being reported.

The present intra-arterial echo catheters fall in three basic categories.

vitro are often reported without such a dome, thus increasing image quality and avoiding the liquid filling process necessary for acoustic coupling.

Rotating element

In Fig. 11, the rotating tip system is schematically illustrated. The shaft (1) must be very flexible and contains the electric wires for the transducer.

The shaft needs to be flexible; yet it must drive the tip in a predictable way. This is nearly impossible when the catheter must follow a tortuous path. As a result, the beam deflection on the display may not correspond with the acoustic beam deflection. This causes errors in the image. Capacitive and optical feed-back techniques have been suggested to cope with this problem. The element (3) is positioned in such a way that no transmission pulse effect appears on the display, since the echo travel time to the dome (2) is of sufficient duration. It allows imaging very close to the catheter outer wall since no 'dead zone' is present. The dome must be acoustically transparent. Results obtained *in-*

Rotating mirror

The rotating mirror technique is similar to the previously described method. Schematically this method is shown in Fig. 12.

The flexible shaft (1); the transparent dome (2); the echotransducer (3) are complemented with a mirror. The mirror creates an even shorter dead zone due to the longer acoustic pathway inside the catheter. The non-moving transducer avoids the necessity of rotating electric wires. Acoustic lenses and focussing shapes of the mirror have been described.

Electronically switched phased array

The catheter shown in Fig. 13 contains many small acoustic elements (2) which are positioned cylindrically around the catheter tip. The number of ele-

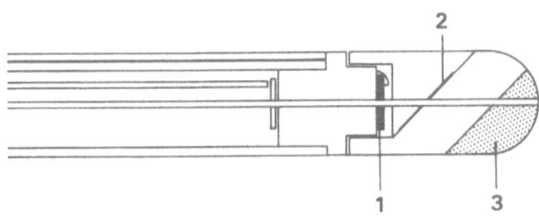

Fig. 10. Echo element (1); rotating mirror (2) and spark erosion electrode (3) as described by Slager [30].

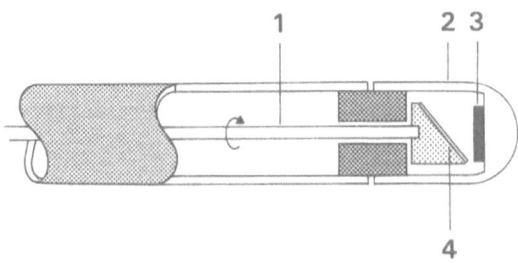

Fig. 12. Mechanically driven echo catheter tip with mirror (4).

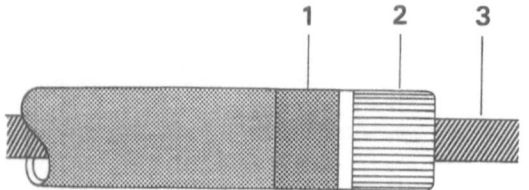

Fig. 13. Electronically switched phased array catheter tip with integrated circuitry for reduction of the number of wires (1); the elements (2) and a guide wire (3).

ments may be any practical number such as 16, 32, 64 or 128. The tip may contain an electronic component to reduce the number of electric wires.

The construction allows for the introduction of a guidewire (3). The principle is identical to the method referred to before (Bom, ref. 20). As illustrated for a small number of rotational symmetric elements in Fig. 14, by introduction of time delays subgroups of elements may together form a

'single larger echo transducer'. This process can be repeated with any other subgroup. In principle this allows aperture variation and electronic focussing methods. On the other hand, acoustic element geometry is not optimal and a near-field dead zone may exist.

Future developments

Intravascular real-time, high resolution ultrasonic imaging is an exciting new development. It produces cross-sectional images of the artery of interest and allows measurement of arterial lumen dimensions extent of atherosclerotic disease. This unique diagnostic potential can be used to characterize the degree of atherosclerotic arterial disease, to grade the effects of pharmacological intervention and to guide angioplasty procedures and evaluate their effects. Of course, combination of

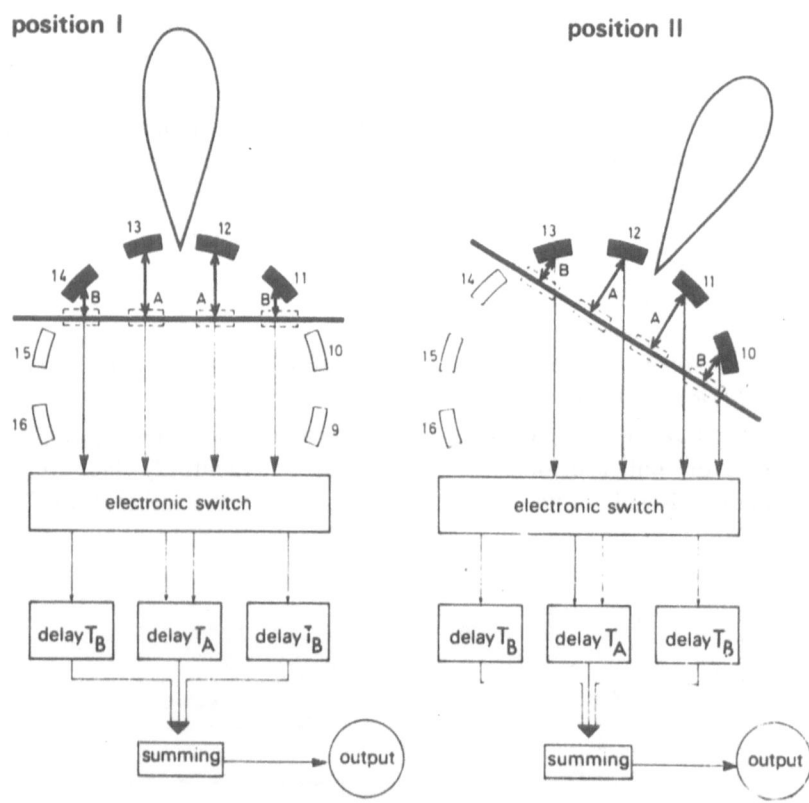

Fig. 14. Principle of phased array catheter tip as described by Bom [20].

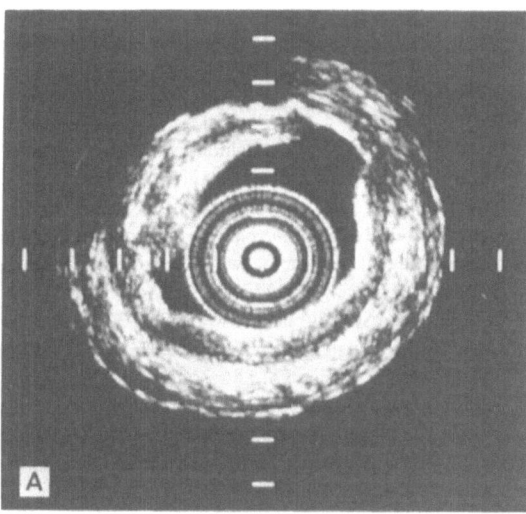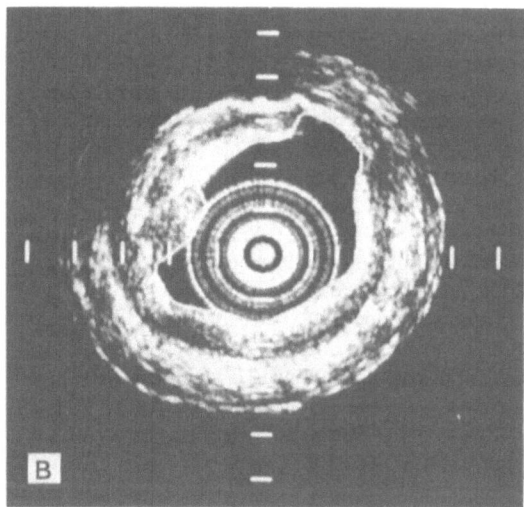

Fig. 15. Echo image as obtained *in vitro* (A) and the automatically derived contour (B); see text.

echography with some of the desobstruction methods will appear in the future. Methods for quantitative evaluation of left ventricular dimensions, as obtained with non-invasive echography, is available today. These quantitative techniques will find their way to analysis of intravascular images as well. An automatic contour analysis for short-axis esophageal echocardiograms based on dynamic programming was developed recently in our laboratory by Bosch [32]. This technique was applied to *in-vitro* vascular images as obtained in Rotterdam. An example is shown in Fig. 15.

This particular image (as shown in Fig. 15A) has been obtained at 32 MHz and clearly shows the particular structures such as plaque and media. The contour obtained with the automatic contour detection technique is shown in Fig. 15B. Thus objective evaluation of a diagnostic situation will become available.

Conclusion

Over the years many attempts to use intraluminal echography have been made. All these ideas from many researchers in the field of diagnostic ultrasound have been a basis for the present developments in intravascular catheter tip echography.

Only when interventional techniques such as PTCA were introduced and thus the clinical need arose, did researchers apply the vast amount of knowledge available to the development of these new exciting devices.

If in the development of echo instrumentation history repeats itself, then the most important clinical application of catheter tip echography will not be the one discussed nowadays.

Acknowledgements

Construction of our catheter prototype has been carried out by Produktcentrum TNO and TPD-TNO at Delft, the Netherlands and the Central Research Workshop of the Erasmus University Rotterdam. The investigations are supported by the Netherlands Technology Foundation (STW) and the Dutch Ministry of Economic Affairs.

References

1. Cieszynski T. Intracardiac method for the investigation of structure of the heart with the aid of ultrasonics. Arch Immun Ter Dow 1960; 8: 551–7.
2. Kossoff G. Diagnostic applications of ultrasound in cardiology. Australas Radiol 1966; X: 101–6.

3. Peronneau P. Catheter with piezoelectric transducer. U.S. Patent No. 3, 542, 014, 1970.

4. Carleton RA, Sessions RW, Graettinger JS. Diameter of heart measured by intracavitary ultrasound. Med Res Engng 1969; May/June: 28–32.

5. Stegall HF, Pratt JR, Moser PF. Carotid mechanics in situ. Fed Proc 1969; 28: 585.

6. Kardon MB, O'Rourke RA, Bishop VS. Measurement of left ventricular internal diameter by catheterization. J Appl Physiol 1971; 31: 613–5.

7. Olson RM, Cooke JP. A nondestructive ultrasonic technique to measure diameter and blood flow in arteries. IEEE Trans Biomed Engng 1974; March: 168–71.

8. Frazin L, Talano JV, Stephanides L, Loeb HS, Kopel L, Gunnar RM. Esophageal echocardiography. Circulation 1976; 54: 102–8.

9. Hughes DJ, Geddes LA, Bourland JD, Babbs CF. Dynamic imaging of the aorta in-vivo with 10 MHz ultrasound. In: Metherell AF, ed. Acoustical imaging 8. New York and London: Plenum Press, 1980: 699–707.

10. Stegall HF, Stone HL, Bishop VS, Laenger C. A catheter-tip pressure and velocity sensor. Proc 20th Ann Conf Eng Med Biol 1967; 27: 4 (abstract).

11. Reid JM, Davis DL, Ricketts HJ, Spencer MP. A new Doppler flowmeter system and its operation with catheter mounted transducers. In: Reneman RS, ed. Cardiovascular applications of ultrasound. Amsterdam/London: North-Holland Publishing Co, 1974: 183–92.

12. Hartley CJ, Cole JS. A single-crystal ultrasonic catheter-tip velocity probe. Med Instrum 1974; 8: 241–3.

13. Sibley DH, Millar HD, Hartley CJ, Whitlow PL. Subselective measurement of coronary blood flow velocity using a steerable Doppler catheter. J Am Coll Cardiol 1986; 8: 1332–40.

14. Gichard FD, Auth DC. Development of a mechanically scanned Doppler blood flow catheter. IEEE Ultrasonics Symp Proc 1975: 306–9.

15. Martin RW, Pollack GH, Phillips J. An ultrasonic catheter tip instrument for measuring volume blood flow. IEEE Ultrasonics Symp Proc 1975: 301–5.

16. Wild JJ, Reid JM. Ultrasonic rectal endoscope for tumor location. Am Inst Ultrasonics Med 1955; 4: 59.

17. Omoto R. Intracardiac scanning of the heart with the aid of ultrasonic intravenous probe. Jap Heart J 8: 569–81.

18. Ebina T, Oka S, Tanaka M, Kosaka S, Kikuchi Y, Uchida R, Hagiwara Y. The diagnostic application of ultrasound to the disease in mediastinal organs. Ultrasono-tomography for the heart and great vessels. Sci Rep Res Inst Tohoku Univ 1965; 12: 199–212.

19. Eggleton RC, Townsend C, Kossoff G, Herrick J, Hunt R, Templeton G, Mitchell JH. Computerised ultrasonic visualization of dynamic ventricular configurations. 8th ICMBE, Palmer House, Chicago IL, July 1969, Session 10–3.

20. Bom N, Lancée CT, Van Egmond FC. An ultrasonic intracardiac scanner. Ultrasonics 1972; 10: 72–6, and US-patent No. 1,402,192, filed February 22, 1973.

21. Hisanaga K, Hisanaga A, Nagata K, Yoshida S. A new transesophageal real-time two-dimensional echocardiographic system using a flexible tube and its clinical application. Proc Jap Soc Ultrasonics Med 1977; 32: 43–4.

22. DiMagno EP, Regan PT, Wilson DA, Buxton JL, Hattery RR, Suarez JR, Green PS. Ultrasonic endoscope. Lancet, March, 1980: 629–31.

23. Bertini A, Masotti L, Zuppiroli A, Cecchi F. Rotating probe for trans-oesophageal cross-sectional echocardiography. J Nucl Med Allied Sci 1984; 28: 115–21.

24. Souquet J, Hanrath P, Zitelli L, Kremer P, Langenstein BA, Schlüter M. Transesophageal phased array for imaging the heart. IEEE Trans Biomed Engng 1982; BME-29: 707–12.

25. Natori H, Tamaki S, Izumi S, Joshita Y, Kira S. Clinical application of ultrasound endoscope using linear array transducer for transesophageal ultrasonography of the disease of the mediastinum. In: Lerski A, Morley P, eds. Ultrasound '82, Oxford: Pergamon Press, 1983: 339–43.

26. Fukuda M. Endoscopic ultrasonography. In: Gill RW, Dadd MJ, eds. WFUMB '85, Sydney/Oxford/New York/Toronto/Frankfurt: Pergamon Press, 1985: 13–6.

27. Nakada A, Matsuo K. An ultrasonic probe for diagnostic examination of the interior body cavities. European patent No. 0 088 620, 1983.

28. Webster WW. Catheter for removing arteriosclerotic plaque. International patent PCT/US84/00474, 1984.

29. Yock PG. Catheter apparatus. European patent No. 0234951, 1987.

30. Slager CJ, Essed CE, Schuurbiers JCH, Bom N, Serruys PW, Meester GT. Vaporization of atherosclerotic plaques by spark erosion. J Am Coll Cardiol 1985; 5: 1382–6.

31. Serruys PW, Jullière Y, Zijlstra F, Beatt KJ, De Feyter PJ, Suryapranata H, Van den Brand M, Roelandt J. Coronary blood flow velocity during percutaneous transluminal coronary angioplasty as guide for assessment of the functional result. Am J Cardiol 1988; 61: 253–9.

32. Bosch JG, Reiber JHC, Van Burken G, Gerbrands JJ, Gussenhoven WJ, Bom N, Roelandt JRTC. Automated endocardial contour detection in short-axis 2-D echocardiograms: methodology and assessment of variability. Proc 15th Int Conf Comp Cardiol 1989 (in press).

International Journal of Cardiac Imaging **4**: 89–97, 1989.

Intraluminal real-time ultrasonic imaging: Clinical perspectives

J. Roelandt & P.W. Serruys
Thoraxcentre, Division of cardiology, University Hospital Rotterdam-Dijkzigt and Erasmus University, Rotterdam, the Netherlands

Introduction

Arteriography with radiological contrast media is currently the principal method for assessment of the presence and severity of both peripheral and coronary vascular disease. The method, however, underestimates the extent and severity of arterial atherosclerotic disease and the large intra- and interobserver variability limits the quantitative assessment of therapeutic interventions [1, 2]. Noninvasive ultrasound imaging provides cross-sectional images of accessible limited portions of the peripheral arterial system [3, 4]. Resolution, however, is limited and the three-layered structure of muscular arteries is rarely appreciated. Precordial cross-sectional echocardiography allows the visualization of proximal parts of the coronary arteries but the success rate is low and the image quality insufficient for clinical decision making in coronary artery disease [5].

The intraoperative epicoronary application of high-frequency ultrasound transducers has confirmed the abnormal findings of earlier pathologic studies and further corroborated the insensitivity of coronary arteriography in appraising the extent and distribution of atherosclerotic wall involvement [6]. Fiberoptic angioscopy allows visualization of the inner surface of the arterial wall and has significantly added to our understanding of the mechanisms of acute ischemic syndromes [7, 8]. The method has practical limitations (it requires complete replacement of blood by large volumes of translucent liquid) and as with contrast arteriography, no information on the arterial wall under the endothelial surface is obtained.

With the rapid progress in interventional radiology and cardiology and more particularly the in-troduction of second-generation therapeutic techniques like mechanical atherectomy and laser, there is an increased risk of vessel perforation. This has stimulated the development of an imaging method to characterize vessel wall pathology and to monitor plaque ablation procedures in real-time, providing the necessary operator feedback on the efficacy of the intervention. Ultrasound offers this potential and has fundamental advantages over all other presently available imaging techniques. Thus, many research groups have directed their efforts to develop ultrasonic real-time intraluminal imaging devices allowing circumferential imaging of the arterial wall under the endothelial surface through the blood. Catheter mounted ultrasound transducers have been used since the early years of cardiac ultrasound in an attempt to improve both sensitivity and image quality by circumventing the limitations inherent in approaching the heart from the chest wall [9–11]. The miniaturization of transducers has led to different approaches for the construction of a miniature catheter-tip based ultrasonic imaging system. At present, single element transducer systems which are either hand-rotated [12] or motor-driven [13–16], and a phased-array system [17], have been developed. It is not clear which of these approaches ultimately will show the optimal design but it may well be that each of these systems may have advantages for a specific application. The study of larger arteries and valve orifices will require lower frequency transducers to be used than those for detailed coronary artery studies. Several groups have published their early experience of both in vitro and in vivo experiments [18–30]. Initial studies have been performed in patients and suggest that intravascular ultrasound imaging is feasible, safe and provides useful clinical information [31–34].

The aim of this contribution is to provide a perspective of the potential research and clinical applications of this exciting new imaging modality (Table 1). Both the specific characteristics of the different intravascular ultrasound imaging catheters and their initial results are extensively described in the different chapters of this book.

Of course, some of these applications are speculative since they are based on experimental rather than clinical information. They fall basically into two categories: diagnosis, and guiding therapeutic interventions. Catheterization of non-vascular small lumina is another potential area of application. These will be mentioned briefly.

Applications in cardiovascular disease

Coronary artery atherosclerosis

Diagnosis, staging and natural history. Intravascular ultrasound imaging shows lumen morphology,

Table 1. Potential applications of intraluminal ultrasound imaging

---

Cardiovascular disease
1. Coronary artery atherosclerosis
   - diagnosis, staging and natural history
   - assessment of therapeutic interventions
     (diet, drugs, catheter based mechanical intervention, coronary bypass surgery, vein graft problems)
2. Peripheral vascular disease
3. Arterial hypertension
   - renal artery stenosis
   - diagnosis and evaluation of treatment
4. Pulmonary arterial disease
5. Valvular heart disease
   - diagnosis of severity
   - valvuloplasty
6. Disease of the aorta
7. Congenital heart disease

Non-cardiovascular disease
1. Urology
2. Obstetrics/gynaecology
3. Gastro-enterology

---

wall micro-architecture, extent of atheroma, and other pathology, and thus offers unique advantages for the diagnosis and treatment of arterial disease. Now, morphometric studies of blood vessels become possible in vivo. In vitro studies have demonstrated the possibility of differentiating between non-calcified fibro-muscular atheroma with fibrosis and lipid deposits, more advanced calcified atheroma, thrombus, plaque rupture and dissection [20, 21, 23–29]. In vitro studies also demonstrate the potential of tissue characterization to provide details of arterial wall pathology [35, 36]. Wall dynamics can be assessed so that the ability of atherosclerotic segments to dilate as a result of vasodilating drugs can be studied [37].

The diagnosis and characterization of arterial atherosclerotic disease offers interesting experimental and clinical possibilities, such as staging its severity and the study of its natural history. Angiography is an insensitive method to assess atherosclerosis. Progress in our understanding of the disease process will be dependent on an imaging method which allows the morphology and composition of the arterial wall to be studied. Recent pathologic studies have further elucidated the atherosclerotic disease process. In its earlier stages, coronary arteries enlarge as a result of a remodelling process of normal segments in relation to plaque area, and functionally important luminal stenosis will not develop until the lesion occupies 40 percent of the circumference of the internal elastic lamina [38]. Thus, serious wall disease may be present despite a nearly normal luminal cross-sectional area on coronary arteriography. The prestenotic phase of atherosclerotic arterial disease in which vascular dysfunction is minimal as previously demonstrated by Armstrong et al. [39] in primates, and confirmed by McPherson et al. [6] with high frequency epicoronary echocardiography during coronary artery bypass surgery in humans. Clearly, identification and characterization of arterial wall involvement is of major interest for research into the natural history of the disease and for attempts to grade its severity. In addition, dynamic rather than static information on the atherosclerotic process can be obtained. Coronary atherosclerosis is a diffuse process, and when the whole artery is diseased, this is seen by echocardiography as diffuse thickening of the arterial wall with reduction in the residual lumen. An example is silent ischemia in patients after cardiac transplantation. Repeated nuclear myocardial perfusion studies and coronary arteriograms are presently used to demonstrate critical lesions as a result of the accelerated progression of atherosclerosis often present in the transplanted heart. In future such diffuse lesions could be assessed quantitatively by intravascular ultrasonic imaging.

Assessment of therapeutic interventions
Cholesterol-lowering diet and drugs. At present, regression studies of atherosclerosis are a major subject for research. Present techniques for studying the degree of atherosclerotic involvement have serious limitations. Quantitative coronary arteriography can be used to define the dimensions of the arterial lumen but it provides no information on the vessel wall and has no value in the early preclinical stages of the disease. In addition, it is tedious and expensive. In more advanced stages of the disease, coronary arteriography reflects only the atheromatous component of the disease process, and provides no information on the sclerosis component or stiffening of the arterial wall [40]. Arterial sclerosis results in reduced systolic expansion and more rapid pulse wave propagation. Pulse wave velocity as well as vessel diameter change can be studied by echo/Doppler techniques [41] but intravascular high resolution real-time ultrasonic imaging would provide more accurate information on systolic wall dynamics. It is conceivable that regression of atherosclerotic wall disease as a result of an intervention would be more successful when started before symptomatic disease is present, and it is unlikely that complex plaques with fibrosis and much calcium will regress with drug therapy. It is therefore important to identify which plaques will regress and which will not. The potential of intravascular imaging techniques to characterize and quantify the disease in its early stages opens exciting perspectives for studying regression of atherosclerosis, whether using a cholesterol-lowering diet of drugs.

Assessment of catheter-based intervention. The number of catheter-based therapeutic interventions for coronary artery stenosis is rapidly increasing, and reached 175,000 procedures in the United States and an estimated 250,000 procedures worldwide in 1987 [42]. An annual increase of approximately 30% is expected [42]. Intravascular ultrasonic imaging would be of major help before, during and after mechanical atherectomy and laser angioplasty as a guidance tool for removing atherosclerotic plaques and deciding the end-point of the intervention [22–30]. Based on detailed information on the wall pathology and its severity, the interventionist may be able to select the most appropriate therapeutic device for a specific lesion.

Fluoroscopy and angioscopy are used to monitor interventions but they have inherent limitations. One of the goals of treatment is to remove as much of the plaque as possible; this could be monitored by an intravascular imaging catheter in order to prevent perforation. Needless to say, much research must be done and much experience must be gained before such information can be used for clinical decision making.

An important clinical question is whether the degree and extent of arterial stenoses (before and after recanalisation procedures) reflect their functional significance. There is ample evidence in the literature that this is not the case [43–45]. Since Doppler catheter systems allow measurement of arterial flow velocity [46], they can be used prior to and after interventions, at rest and following pharmacologically induced maximal vasodilatation, to assess the functional significance of the original and any remaining stenosis [47, 48]. The potential combination of measurement of arterial cross-sectional area by the imaging technique and blood flow velocity by the Doppler technique would improve our understanding of coronary artery disease and further help to assess the results of intervention.

The angiographic appearance of the post-intervention region is often suboptimal for interpretation of the result and does not allow to predict acute and chronic complications. The presence and severity of dissection of the wall may be visualized directly, and could be used to develop criteria for stent implantation (Fig. 1). Morphologic criteria may be established which predict acute or chronic restenosis, which is the major problem of balloon angioplasty since it occurs in up to 30% of patients.

Coronary bypass surgery. Intravascular ultrasonic imaging allows intraoperative evaluation of the anastomosis between vein grafts or internal mammary arteries and the native coronary arteries. By measuring the width of the opening and the presence of atheroma at the anastomosis, the adequacy of the graft can be evaluated. Intraoperative epicoronary studies by Hiratzka [49] have demonstrated that end-to-side anastomoses tend to have a larger anastomotic opening than side-to-side anastomoses. Potentially, intravascular high-frequency ultrasonic imaging yields images of the anastomotic site with better resolution and detail than epicoronary high frequency imaging. Predisposition of bypass grafts to close may be related to the condition of the vessel wall and the surgical results of the anastomosis. Information could also be obtained to decide upon endarterectomy, and the technique has the potential to control the result of this procedure. It could also be used to study the mechanisms of platelet deposition, neointimal proliferation and graft atherosclerosis in venous bypass grafts in vivo.

Peripheral vascular disease

Contrast angiography remains the principal method for the evaluation of patients with symptomatic peripheral vascular disease. Once the angiographic information is available, either surgery or percutaneous transluminal angioplasty (PTA) which is a much less complex, less invasive and a less expensive procedure, is performed [50]. During the PTA procedure, detailed information about the arterial wall allows the appropriate intervention procedure to be chosen (laser, balloon atherectomy) and the correct balloon size to be selected when the stenosis can be passed. The result of the therapeutic procedure can be verified immediately and measured quantitatively [22, 26, 30]. Maximal plaque ablation could result in a lower restenosis rate and too much thinning of the arterial wall with risk of aneurysm formation could be avoided [28]. At pre-

sent, intraoperative angiography is still being performed to assess the result in approximately half of the patients undergoing peripheral vascular surgery. Fiberoptic angioscopy has been used but has practical limitations both after PTA and surgery. Although it provides detailed images of the lumen and the endothelial surface, it did not avoid perforation during peripheral laser angioplasty in 55% of the patients where it was used as guidance tool [51]. The ultrasonic guidance and assessment of PTA procedures opens the prospect of outpatient endovascular surgical procedures.

Much of our present knowledge of carotid artery atherosclerosis is based on external ultrasound examination and duplex scanning. Angiography is now being more and more displaced as the primary method for the evaluation of patients prior to carotid endarterectomy. In addition to the severity of stenosis, the type of plaque can be assessed by ultrasound and may be predictive of the risk of stroke [52]. The potential role of intravascular ultrasound imaging both for the diagnosis of carotid artery disease and to assist during carotid endarterectomy is difficult to predict.

Arterial hypertension

It has been known for more than a century that the walls of arteries are thickened in patients with arterial hypertension. Research in studying the arterial wall has been limited because of the lack of a reliable method to obtain quantitative data about the arterial wall. Increased wall thickness and more particularly media thickness/lumen diameter ratio have been documented by measurements from pathological specimens. When arterioles of patients with hypertension were compared to arterioles from matched normals, a 29% increase in media thickness/lumen diameter ratio was found [53]. The question is whether this structural abnormality is a consequence or the cause of the hypertension. This important question could be studied prospectively with the ultrasound catheter. Intravascular imaging allows the accurate measurement of media thickness/lumen diameter, the resolution of ultrasound imaging systems being approximately 75 microns. The first question which should be answered is whether media thickening present in medium sized arteries such as the femoral and brachial arteries parallels the medial hypertrophy of the arterioles. Other new directions for studying arterial hypertension include grading of the severity of the disease, and whether (and which) antihypertensive medication reverses structural wall changes. It has been shown in experimental studies that this indeed occurs with some drugs [54]. The influence of antihypertensive treatment on atherosclerosis-related complications is another potential research area.

Renal artery stenosis is the cause of arterial hypertension in 5–10% of patients, and results from atherosclerosis or fibromuscular dysplasia. Percutaneous transluminal renal angioplasty has already become the treatment of choice because of its advantages over surgery and antihypertensive drug treatment, which may not halt the progressive deterioration in kidney function. In addition, some stenotic intrarenal arterial segments may be inaccessible to surgery, and angioplasty would then be the method of choice. Here too, intravascular ultrasound imaging may offer advantages for guiding the procedure and assess the results.

Pulmonary arterial disease

Unfortunately, the transition from elastic to muscular type of artery occurs very distal in the pulmonary circulation and assessment of the resistance (muscular) arteries is impossible with presently available size of catheters. Nevertheless, intimal fibrosis, atherosclerosis and chronic thromboembolic pulmonary disease may be evaluated by the ultrasound imaging catheter.

Valvular heart disease

Potential applications are the real-time imaging of valve morphology and function. Measurement of valve orifice area in patients with valvular heart disease would be possible [55]. The method can be used for measuring orifice area before and after balloon valvulotomy. Mitral valve disease results in increased pulmonary venous pressure. In long-standing cases medial hypertrophy develops known as 'arterialization' of the pulmonary veins [56]. Measurement of pulmonary vein hypertrophy could help to assess and predict the reversibility of pulmonary hypertension as a result of mitral valve disease.

Diseases of the aorta

Lumen geometry and other characteristics of the aortic wall can be recorded, thereby allowing the study of atherosclerotic involvement and its complications. Transesophageal echocardiography provides information on the thoracic aorta but not on the abdominal aorta. This is possible with the ultrasound imaging catheter and may offer advantages for the complete evaluation of acute aortic dissection in some patients. Coarctation of the aorta is another condition in which a direct quantitative assessment is possible.

Congenital heart disease

One could easily speculate about the potential of intracavitary and intravascular imaging in newborns and infants. Initial feasibility studies have shown that high resolution images of cardiac structures can be obtained [57]. The device also permits transesophageal echocardiographic imaging in newborns and infants. The imaging catheter could be used to select balloon size and assess morphology before and after dilatation of aortic coarctation or peripheral pulmonary arterial stenosis. The suitability of both the pulmonary and aortic valve for balloon valvuloplasty are other potential applications. In newborns and infants, anomalous venous connections are difficult to diagnose by precordial echocardiography or by angiocardiography, but could be visualized from within the right atrium.

Applications in non-cardiovascular disease

Urology

Prostate cancer is, after lung cancer, the most common cause of death from malignant disease in males. Transrectal ultrasonic scanning of the prostate is being used for the detection of the early stages of cancer which are curable, but this approach and other diagnostic methods have both limited sensitivity and specificity. Transurethral ultrasound imaging may offer the potential of a superior diagnostic method to detect prostate cancer in situ.

Ureteric cancers are rare and often infiltrating. Because adequate diagnostic methods to diagnose spread of these tumors into the submucosal and muscular layers of the ureter are not available, there is an inappropriate number of unneccesary surgical procedures. Catheterisation of the ureter with fiberoptic catheters is now routine practice, and the use of a 5F high-frequency ultrasonic imaging system would be no problem and could provide important information.

Obstetrics/gynaecology

Catheterisation with the small-sized high resolution imaging catheter of the corpus uteri and Fallopian tubes is possible extending diagnostic capabilities by obtaining information from submucosal structures. In early pregnancy it may allow the study of early embryonic development.

Gastro-enterology

Endoscopic procedures of the gastro-intestinal tract are becoming more and more sophisticated, and endoscopic retrograde cholangio-pancreatography (ERCP) is being used increasingly to detect and diagnose gall bladder, duct and pancreatic disease. The ultrasound imaging catheter could become an adjunct to ERCP procedures in selected patients.

Factors influencing image quality and interpretation

The interpretation of arterial cross-sectional images is not always straightforward as a result of physical factors influencing image quality (Table 2). Proper alignment of the catheter in the long axis is necessary to obtain adequate images of the arterial wall. The perpendicularity of the ultrasound beam to the wall structures influences the intensity of these structures on the display, and minor angular changes have significant effects. Differentiation between structures and pathologic changes based on their intensity on the display may be ambiguous. Similar problems arise from the proximity effect as there is rapid attenuation of ultrasound energy with distance to the vessel wall. Eccentric positioning results in high intensity echoes of the adjacent wall structures which appear thicker, while similar structures in the opposite more distant wall appear hypoechoic.

Inadequate resolution is another cause of ambiguous results. The scanning ultrasound beam rapidly increases in width with distance and when highly reflective abnormalities such as areas of calcification are present at the edge of the beam, they may be projected into the imaging plane, falsely suggesting fibrosis in that area.

Future perspectives

Initial research has been devoted to combining the intraluminal imaging device with ablation techniques such as spark erosion [58]. The combination of imaging with an ultrasound angioplasty technique would be another exciting possibility [59]. The diagnostic potential also includes tissue characterisation capabilities and this possibility has al-

Table 2. Physical factors influencing image quality

- Catheter alignment to vessel wall
- Perpendicularity of wall structures
- Attenuation due to distance
- Beam width/lateral resolution

ready been shown in vitro [35, 36]. This combination could be of further help as a guidance tool. Intracoronary Doppler flow velocity measurements prior to and after interventions are now being used to assess the result of the procedure [47, 48].

The combination of measurement of arterial cross-sectional area by catheter-tip imaging, and blood flow velocimetry would certainly improve such assessments and allow distal run-off to be measured. The additional simultaneous measurement of pressure within the artery would allow the determination of pressure-volume relationships and stiffness of that particular segment of the vessel wall. Three-dimensional reconstructions of postmortem arterial specimens and of segments of the femoral artery in vivo have already been realized [60], and further increase the capabilities of plaque quantification, both in extent and volume. A major help during second generation ablation techniques (laser, spark erosion, mechanical atherectomy) would be the development of an imaging system which can look forwards from rather than orthogonal to the catheter.

Conclusion

Intravascular, real-time, high-resolution echography is an exciting new development. It produces circumferential images of the artery segment of interest and allows measurement of lumen dimensions, wall thickness and extent of wall disease. This unprecedented diagnostic potential opens new horizons for clinical research and practical applications are rapidly emerging. It can be used to characterise and quantify the degree of arterial

Table 3. Future perspectives

- Combination with ablation techniques
- Combination with pressure measurement
- Combination with Doppler velocimetry
- Three-dimensional reconstruction
- Tissue characterisation
- Forward (down-stream) imaging

disease, to study its natural history, and to grade the effects of pharmacologic interventions. It will become a major adjunct to second-generation angioplasty procedures, as a guidance tool and for the immediate evaluation of results, since it is more easy to use and provides unique information much faster than other imaging modalities.

References

1. Fisher LD, Judkins MP, Lesperance J, et al. Reproducibility of coronary arteriographic reading in the coronary artery surgery study (CASS). Cathet Cardiovasc Diag 1982; 8: 565–75.
2. Siegel RJ, Swan K, Edwalds G, et al. Limitations of postmortem assessment of human coronary artery size and luminal narrowing: differential effects of tissue fixation and processing on vessels with different degrees of atherosclerosis. J Am Coll Cardiol 1985; 5: 342–6.
3. Pignoli P, Tremoli HE, Poli A, et al. Intimal plus medial thickness of the arterial wall: a direct measurements with ultrasound imaging. Circulation 1986; 74: 1399–406.
4. Blankenhorn DH, Chin HP, Conover DJ, et al. Ultrasound observation on pulsation in human carotid artery lesions. Ultrasound in Med & Biol 1988; 14, 7: 583–7.
5. Taams MA, Gussenhoven EJ, Cornel JH, et al. Detection of left coronary artery stenosis by transoesophageal echocardiography. Eur Heart J 1988; 9: 1162–66.
6. McPherson DD, Hiratzka LF, Lamberth WC, et al. Delineation of the extent of coronary atherosclerosis by high-frequency epicardial. N Engl J Med 1987; 316: 304–9.
7. Forrester JS, Litvack F, Grundfest W, et al. A Perspective of coronary disease seen through the arteries of living man. Circulation 1987; 75: 505.
8. Forrester JS, Litvack F, Grundfest W, et al. Cardiac angioscopy in acute ischemic syndromes. Am J Card Imaging 1988; 2: 178–84.
9. Wild JJ, Reid JM. Progress in techniques of soft tissue examination by 15 MC pulsed ultrasound. In: Kelly E (ed) Ultrasound in Medicine and Biology, Washington, American Institute of Biological Sciences, 1950; p. 30.
10. Cieszynski T. Intracardiac method for the investigation of structure of the heart with the aid of ultrasonics. Arch Immun Ter Dosw 1960; 8: 551–7.
11. Kimoto S, Omoto R, Tsunemoto M, et al. Ultrasonic tomography of the liver and detection of heart atrial septal defect with the aid of ultrasonic intravenous probes. Ultrasonics 1964; 2: 82–6.
12. Mallery JA, Gregory K, Morcos NC, et al. Evaluation of an ultrasound balloon dilatation imaging catheter. Circulation 1987; 76: IV–371 (Abstr).
13. Yock PG, Linker DT, Thapliyal HV, et al. Real-time, two-dimensional catheter ultrasound: a new technique for

high-resolution intravascular imaging. J Am Coll Cardiol 1988; 11: 130 A (abstr).

14. Bom N, Lancee CT, Slager CJ, et al. Ein Weg zur intraluminaren Echoarteriographie. Ultraschall 1987; 8: 233–6.

15. Pandian NG, Kreis A, Brockway B, et al. Ultrasound angioscopy: real-time, two-dimensional, intraluminal ultrasound imaging of blood vessels. Am J Cardiol 1988; 62: 493–4.

16. Roelandt JR, Bom N, Serruys PW, et al. Intravascular high-resolution real-time cross-sectional echocardiography. Echocardiography 1989; 6: 1–8.

17. Hodgson J, Eberle MJ, Savakus MD, et al. Validation of a new real time percutaneous intravascular ultrasound imaging catheter. Circulation 1988; 78: II–21 (abstr).

18. Mallery JA, Griffith J, Gessert J, et al. Intravascular ultrasound imaging catheter assessment of normal and atherosclerotic arterial wall thickness. J Am Coll Cardiol 1988; II: 22A (abstr). 18.

19. Gussenhoven WJ, Bom N, van Egmond FC, et al. A high frequency ultrasound catheter for intravascular imaging. Eur Heart J 1988; 9: 802 (abstr).

20. Pandian N, Kreis A, O'Donnell T, et al. Intraluminal two-dimensional ultrasound angioscopic quantitation of arterial stenosis: comparison with external high frequency ultrasound imaging and anatomy. J Am Coll Cardiol 1989; 13: 5A (abstr).

21. Pandian N, Kreis A, Brockway B, et al. Detection of intravascular thrombus by high frequency intraluminal ultrasound angioscopy: in vitro and in vivo studies. J Am Coll Cardiol 1989; 13: 5A (abstr).

22. Mallery JA, Mahon D, Griffith J, et al. Intravascular ultrasound visualization of atheroma plaque removal by atherectomy. J Am Coll Cardiol 1989; 13: 222A (abstr).

23. Roelandt JR, Serruys PW, Bom N, et al. Intravascular real-time high resolution two-dimensional echocardiography. J Am Coll Cardiol 1989; 13: 4A (abstr).

24. Bartorelli AL, Potkin BN, Almagor Y, et al. Intravascular ultrasound imaging of atherosclerotic coronary arteries: an in vitro validation study. J Am Coll Cardiol 1989; 13: 4A (abstr).

25. Gussenhoven WJ, Essed CE, Lancee CT, et al. Arterial wall characteristics determined by intravascular ultrasound imaging: an in vitro study. J Am Coll Cardiol (in press).

26. Pandian N, Kreis A, Brockway B, et al. Intraluminal ultrasound angioscopic detection of arterial dissection and intimal flaps: in vitro and vivo studies. Circulation 1988; 78: II–21 (abstr).

27. Mallery JA, Tobis JM, Gessert J, et al. Evaluation of an intravascular ultrasound imaging catheter in porcine peripheral and coronary arteries in vivo. Circulation 1988; 78: II–21 (abstr).

28. Yock PG, Johnson EL, Linker DT. Intravascular ultrasound: development and clinical potential. Am J Card Imaging 1988; 2: 185–93.

29. Mallery JA, Tobis JM, Gessert J, et al. Identification of tissue components in human atheroma by an intravascular ultrasound imaging catheter. Circulation 1988; 78, 4: II–22 (abstr).

30. Graham SP, Brands D, Savakus A, et al. Utility of an intravascular ultrasound imaging device for arterial wall definition and atherectomy guidance. J Am Coll Cardiol 1989; 13: 222A (abstr).

31. Yock P, Linker D, Seather D, et al. Intravascular two-dimensional catheter ultrasound: initial clinical studies. Circulation 1988; 78: II–21 (abstr).

32. Meyer CR, Chiang EH, Fechner KP, et al. Feasibility of high-resolution intravascular ultrasonic imaging catheter. Radiology 1988; 168: 113–6.

33. Pandian N, Kreis A, Desnoyers M, et al. In vivo ultrasound angioscopy in humans and animals: intraluminal imaging of blood vessels using a new catheter-based high resolution ultrasound probe. Circulation 1988; 78: II–22 (abstr).

34. Hodgson J, Graham SP, Savakus A. Percutaneous intravascular ultrasound imaging in humans: initial peripheral and coronary studies. Proceedings 4th Intl Congress on Cardiac Doppler, Anaheim, 1989.

35. Linker DT, Yock PG, Thapliyal HV, et al. In vitro analysis of back scattered amplitude from normal and diseased arteries using a new intraluminal ultrasonic catheter. J Am Coll Cardiol 1988; 11: 4A (abstr).

36. Martinelli MA, Aretz TH, Butterly J. Ultrasonic imaging of coronary arterial thickness and ultrasonic signature typing of internal abnormalities. In: Microsensors and Catheter-based Imaging Technology. Alan I. West (ed), Proc. SPIE 1988; 904: 110–5.

37. McPherson DD, Ross AF, Moyers JR, et al. Can atherosclerotic coronaries vasodilate? An intraoperative high-frequency epicardial echocardiographic study. Circulation 1986; 74: II–468 (abstr).

38. Glagov S, Weisenberg E, Zarins CK, et al. Compensatory enlargement of human atherosclerotic arteries. N Engl J Med 1987; 316: 1371–5.

39. Armstrong ML, Heistad DD, Marcus ML, et al. Structural and hemodynamic responses of peripheral arteries of macaque monkeys to atherogenic diet. Atherosclerosis 1985; 5: 336–46.

40. Blankenhorn DH, Krausch DM. Reversal of atherosclerosis and sclerosis: the two components of atherosclerosis. Circulation 1989; 79: 1–7.

41. Levenson JA, Simon AC, Maarik BE, et al. Regional compliance of brachial artery and saline infusion in patients with arteriosclerosis obliteraus. Atherosclerosis 1985; 5: 80–7.

42. Bourassa MG, Alderman EL, Bertrand M, et al. Report of the joint ISFC/WHO Task force on coronary angioplasty. Circulation 1988; 78: 780–9.

43. Marcus M, Wright C, Doty D, et al. Measurements of coronary velocity and reactive hyperemia in the coronary circulation of humans. Circ Res 1981; 49: 877–91.

44. Harrison DG, White CW, Hiratzka LF, et al. Can the significance of coronary stenosis be predicted by quantitative coronary angiography? Circulation 1981; 64: 160 (abstr).

45. White CW, Wright CW, Doty DB, et al. Does visual interpretation of the coronary arteriogram predict the physiologic importance of a coronary stenosis? N Engl J Med 1984; 310: 819–24.

46. Cole JS, Hartley CJ. The pulsed Doppler coronary artery catheter: preliminary report of a new technique for measuring rapid changes in coronary artery flow velocity in man. Circulation 1977; 56: 18–25.

47. Serruys PW, Zijlstra F, Reiber JHC, et al. Assessment of coronary flow reserve during angioplasty using a Doppler tip balloon catheter. Comparison with digital subtraction cineangiography. J Interven Cardiol 1988; 1: 19–33.

48. Serruys PW, Julliere Y, Zijlstra F, et al. Coronary blood flow velocity during percutaneous transluminal coronary angioplasty as a guide for assessment of the functional result. Am J Cardiol 1988; 61: 253–59.

49. Hiratzka LF, McPherson DD, Lamberth WC, et al. Intraoperative evaluation of coronary artery bypass graft anastomoses with high-frequency epicardial echocardiography: experimental validation and initial patient studies. Circulation 1986; 73: 1199–205.

50. Doubilet P, Abrams HL. The cost of underutilization percutaneous transluminal angioplasty for peripheral vascular disease. N Engl J Med 1983; 310: 25–102.

51. Abela GS, Seeger JM, Barbieri, et al. Laser angioplasty with angioscopic guidance in humans. J Am Coll Cardiol 1986; 8: 184–92.

52. Reilly LM, Lusby RJ, Hughes L, et al. Carotid plaque histology using real-time ultrasonography. Clinical and therapeutic implications. Am J Surg 1983; 146: 188–93.

53. Aalkjaer C, Heagerty AM, Petersen KK, et al. Evidence for increased media thickness, increased neuronal amine uptake and depressed excitation-contraction coupling in isolated resistance vessels from essential hypertensives. Circ Res 1987; 61: 181–6.

54. Owens GK. Influence of blood pressure on development of aortic medial smooth muscle hypertrophy in spontaneously hypertensive rats. Hypertension 1987; 9: 179–87.

55. Heldman D, Mallery J, Spear G, et al. Intravascular ultrasound imaging catheter accurately measures area of stenotic aortic valves in vitro. J Am Coll Cardiol 1983; 13, 2: 49A (abstr).

56. Wagenvoort CA. Morphologic changes in the intrapulmonary veins. Human Pathology 1970; 1: 205–13.

57. Valdes-Cruz L, Sahn DJ, Yock P, et al. Experimental animal investigations of the potential for new approaches to diagnostic cardiac imaging in infants and small premature infants from intracardiac and transesophageal approaches using a 20 MHz real time ultrasound imaging catheter. J Am Coll Cardiol 1989; 13, 2: 137A (abstr).

58. Bom N, Slager CJ, Van Egmond FC, et al. Intra-arterial ultrasonic imaging for recanalization by spark erosion. Ultrasound Med Biol 1988; 14: 257–61.

59. Freeman I, Isner JM, Gal D, et al. Ultrasonic angioplasty using a new flexible wire system. J Am Coll Cardiol 1989; 13, 2: 4A (abstr).

60. Kitney RI, Moura L, Straughan K, et al. Three dimensional solid modelling of arterial structures using ultrasound. Proc IEEE IXth Conf on Engng Med & Biol 1987; 400–13.

International Journal of Cardiac Imaging **4**: 99–104, 1989.

Ultrasound imaging and atherogenesis

A.E. Becker
Department of Pathology, Academic Medical Center, Meibergdreef 9, 1105 AZ Amsterdam-Zuidoost, The Netherlands

Abstract

The in vivo detection of early atherosclerosis remains a problem. First, atherogenesis is a process with an insidious onset and course. Once clinical signs and symptoms have developed the lesion usually is in an advanced stage. Second, the detection of early atherosclerotic lesions creates the problem of distinguishing between almost natural, age-related intimal changes and intimal thickening as a precursor lesion of atherosclerosis. The hallmark of atherosclerosis is the abnormal deposition of lipids within the intima. This process is accompanied by a cellular response, composed of macrophages, lymphocytes and proliferating vascular smooth muscle cells. An increasing quantity of collagen and elastin fibers eventually will replace the cellular constituents. In other words, a changing histological picture with respect to component make up in time. Third, an adequate interpretation of intimal thickening may be complicated further by tissue characteristics of the arterial media. The elastin units of an elastic type artery produce an echo-dense image, whereas a muscular media is hypoechoic. All in all it seems fair to state that ultrasound imaging techniques, at least for the time being, will be inadequate to distinguish between 'early' atherosclerotic lesions and intimal thickenings which will not necessarily progress to the full blown lesion.

Introduction

Ultrasound imaging techniques have developed to the extent that in vivo tissue characterization is no longer utopia. As an immediate spin off of these technological assessments the question arises whether or not ultrasound techniques may be used for the detection of early atherosclerosis. This brings into discussion the mechanisms involved in atherogenesis, the definition of an atherosclerotic lesion, the tissue component make up of such lesions, the histological changes that may occur in time and the tissue characteristics of the arteries involved.

Atherosclerotic lesions: A matter of definition

In previous days atherosclerosis usually was described as a disease, affecting arteries and charac-
terized by a thickening of the intima, composed mainly of fatty debris embedded within dense collagen tissue and often further complicated by extensive calcific deposits (Fig. 1). It is presently well accepted that this image of the atherosclerotic lesion represents an 'end-stage disease' which has developed over a long period of time. Nevertheless, from a clinical viewpoint this is the lesion associated with major clinical events, such as myocardial infarction. This discrepancy once more highlights the problem that the arterial disease has an insidious onset and course and becomes evident only because of the occurence of secondary, clinical signs and symptoms. Usually, the underlying atherosclerotic lesion then has been complicated by a plaque fissure and localized occlusive thrombosis or by thromboembolic events. Important facets as far as treatment and prognosis are concerned, but of little relevance when it comes to the recognition of the disease prior to its clinical stage.

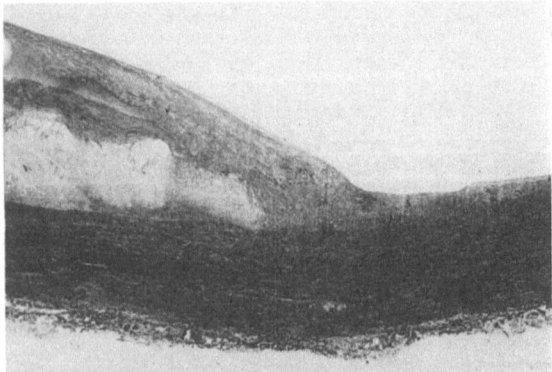

Fig. 1. Micrograph of 'classical' atherosclerosis. There is intimal thickening with a central core of atheromatous debris surrounded by dense connective tissue, almost a-cellular. Elastic tissue stain.

Having established the need for early detection of atherosclerosis the question arises whether or not 'early' lesions are clearly defined. In this arena much controversy still lingers [1]. One of the earliest changes to occur in arteries is the development of a musculo-elastic layer within the intima (Fig. 2). Smooth muscle cells, most likely derived from the media, proliferate and migrate into the intima and produce matrix substances which eventually differentiate into recognizable connective tissue elements [2]. With the increase in age this layer gradually transforms into a fiborus layer without much cellularity, and is known as 'diffuse intimal thickening'. This transitional phenomenon, together with changes in the media, is generally referred to as 'arteriosclerosis of the elderly'.

The question thus arises is diffuse intimal thickening a precursor lesion for atherosclerosis? The answer is probably no, unless additional circumstances are present that promote lipid accumulation (see below). Indeed the hallmark of the atherosclerotic lesion still is a pathological accumulation of lipids, within the intima, in conjunction with a tissue response. This may occur in an otherwise unaffected intima (as for instance in many of the experimental animal models) or in an already altered intima, as previously outlined. This does not imply that lipids already should have accumulated into distinct atheromatous pools, but their presence in abnormal quantities is essential to des-

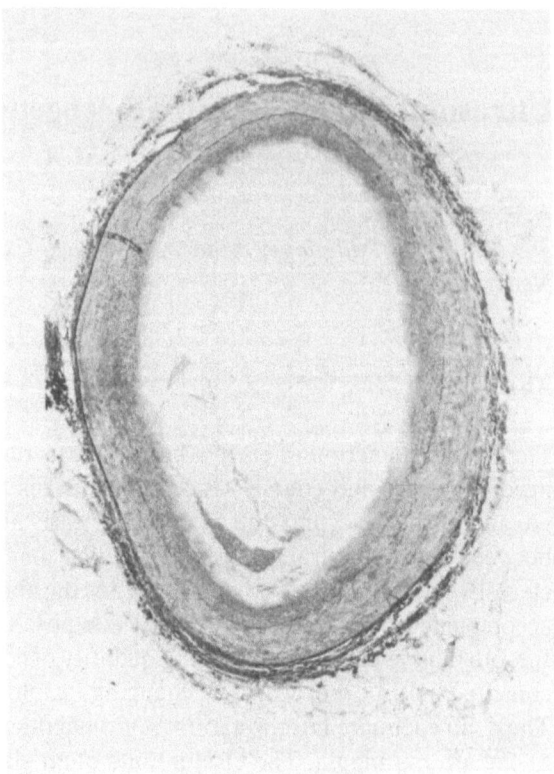

Fig. 2. Micrograph showing a cross section through a coronary artery with a distinct musculo-elastic layer, causing intimal thickening. This layer is composed of smooth muscle cells intermingled with collagen and elastin fibers and lacks the almost circular orientation of the smooth muscle cells in the media. Elastic tissue stain.

ignate the change as an 'atherosclerotic lesion'. This then creates the problem to identify lesions which do contain lipids, but not necessarily as atheromatous debris.

Atherogenesis: Basic mechanisms

The precise mechanisms involved in atherogenesis are as yet not fully understood. Nevertheless, much insight has been accumulated over the past decades, particularly with respect to the early stages of this disease.

It is presently acknowledged that atherogenesis is directly related to dysfunction of endothelial cells. For a long period of time the latter have been considered as a simple barrier between blood and tissue components of the arterial wall. This concept has been changed drastically over the past decades [3]. The endothelial cells play an active role in prohibiting injurious tissue effects of blood borne 'unfriendly' agents. In this context the selective barrier function with respect to lipoproteins may be crucial. Indeed, an active transport of lipids over the endothelial cell layer is taking place and may be one of the keys to an understanding of early athero-genesis. A disturbance in the normal endothelial 'barrier' function, for instance because of harmful effects of changes in shear stress or due to high plasma levels of lipoproteins, could induce an ex-cessive influx of lipids into the intima. Monocytes may penetrate the intima, transform into tissue macrophages and phagocytose lipids. However, once lipids accumulate in excess, macrophages may no longer be able to clear the tissues.

The cells may desintegrate exposing free radicals to the tissue, thus enhancing further injury. More-over, macrophages may produce a potent growth factor, that may induce proliferation, and probably migration, of vascular smooth muscle cells. Im-mune phenotyping of these cells show them to ex-press a synthetic nature, as judged from a shift in the vimentin-desmin ratio. A phenomenon gener-ally considered as an expression of the potential capability of such cells to produce matrix substanc-es and, hence, fibrous tissues. Moreover, activated T lymphocytes occur in close contact with macro-phages, thus suggesting an immune-mediated re-sponse [4].

Once set into pace one may conceptualize that a sequence of events is introduced that ultimately may lead to an elevated lesion in which lipids and a fibrocellular tissue response dominate the picture. However, the precise composition may vary con-siderably, particularly in time.

Atherosclerosis: Component make up variability

Studying atherosclerotic lesions it is obvious that the component make up differs markedly from one site to the other in a given artery, from one location to the other within the same lesion and from one artery to the other in a given patient. In other

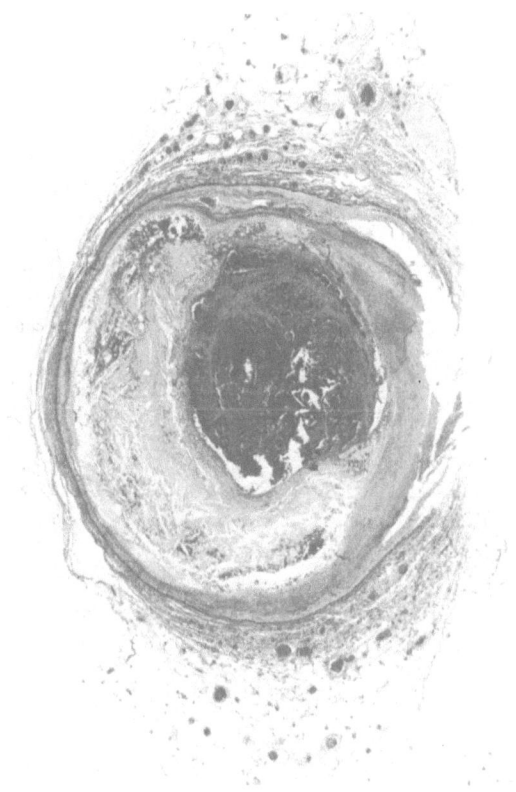

Fig. 3. Micrograph showing an atherosclerotic lesion almost solely composed of atheromatous debris. Elastic tissue stain.

words, there is no such thing as a uniform plaque, other than that lesions do fit within a common basic framework.

In some instances the lesion is dominated by the atheroma, that is the pool of lipids with cellular debris as 'leftover' of attempts to remove the infil-tration of fat (Fig. 3). In other instances, the lesion is dominated by fibrous tissue with only a minimal amount of atheromatous debris (Fig. 4). This im-plies that the cells, such as macrophages and lym-phocytes have largely disappeared and that the vascular smooth muscle cells have transformed the cellular lesion into a mainly collagenous one [5]. If one accepts this as a gradual transition in time, it also implies that various stages of atherosclerotic lesions should be encountered with quantitative differences in component make up.

It is accepted, also, that the differences in com-ponent make up of atherosclerotic plaque reflects in the probability of complications. A difference

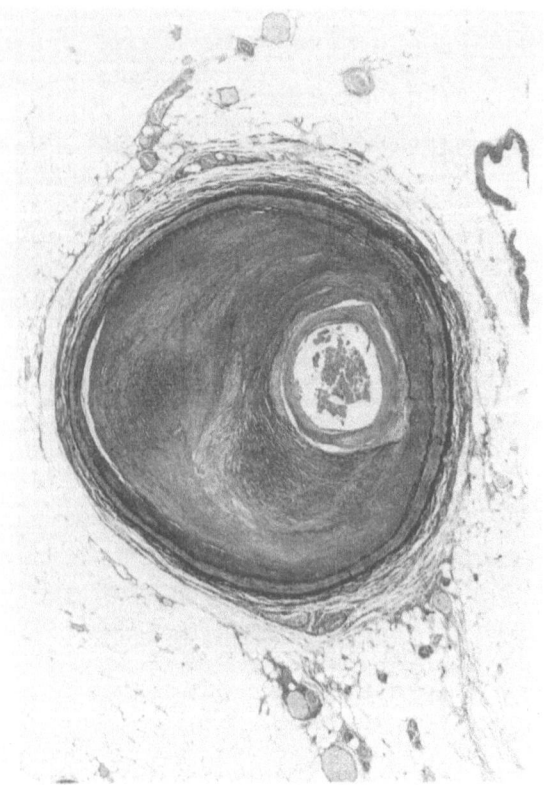

Fig. 4. Micrograph showing a cross section through a coronary artery with an atherosclerotic lesion almost solely composed of fibrous tissue. Elastic tissue stain.

has been proposed between so-called plaques at risk and those not at risk.

Plaques at risk are those in which the atheromatous debris is protected from the lumen by a thin, and often tethered fibrotic cap only. The atheroma, therefore, is almost directly exposed to the lumen. From this observation one may hypothesize that hemodynamic changes can induce surface alterations that lead to complications such as platelet aggregation and thrombus formation. Similarly, since the muscular media in most arteries with advanced atherosclerotic lesions is intact, vasocontraction still could occur. In fact this phenomenon is accepted generally as *the* underlying mechanism of a 'cracked' plaque and the almost inevitable thrombotic complication.

Atherosclerosis and arteries: Tissue characteristics

Atherosclerotic lesions occur in large, elastic arteries such as the aorta and proximal segments of the carotid and iliac arteries, and middle-sized muscular arteries. As far as presently known there is no major difference in the intima and its endothelial cell coating between both types. However, the media is the distinctive layer. Elastic arteries show a media composed of functional units, themselves formed by smooth muscle cells, matrix substances and collagen and elastin fibers, sandwiched between two elastin lamellae (Fig. 5). The number of units may vary considerably. In the thoracic aorta the number of units is higher than in the abdominal aorta below the level of the origin of the renal arteries.

Muscular arteries, on the other hand, do not contain this lamellar composition of the media. The latter is almost solely composed of smooth muscle cells with sparse collagen and elastin fibers in between (Fig. 6). It should be emphasized, in this context, that the amount of collagen and elastin varies. With increasing age the amount of connective tissue increases also. This, together with fibrous changes within the intima, may have considerable impact on ultrasound imaging [6]. Another important feature that relates to the muscular media is the spatial orientation of the smooth muscle cells. It is generally propagated that the smooth muscle cells are arranged in circular fashion. In reality, however, the cells form a helix, often with a different curve at different levels.

Atherosclerosis: Ultrasound imaging

From the point of view of ultrasound imaging of atherosclerotic lesions it is of the utmost significance that no uniformity exists with respect to tissue component make up. Once the lesion has reached an advanced stage, for instance causing excessive luminal obstruction, the precise component make up may not be what the ultrasound tissue identification method is able to detect. The thickness of the lesion and its location within the artery may be satisfactory visualized and these

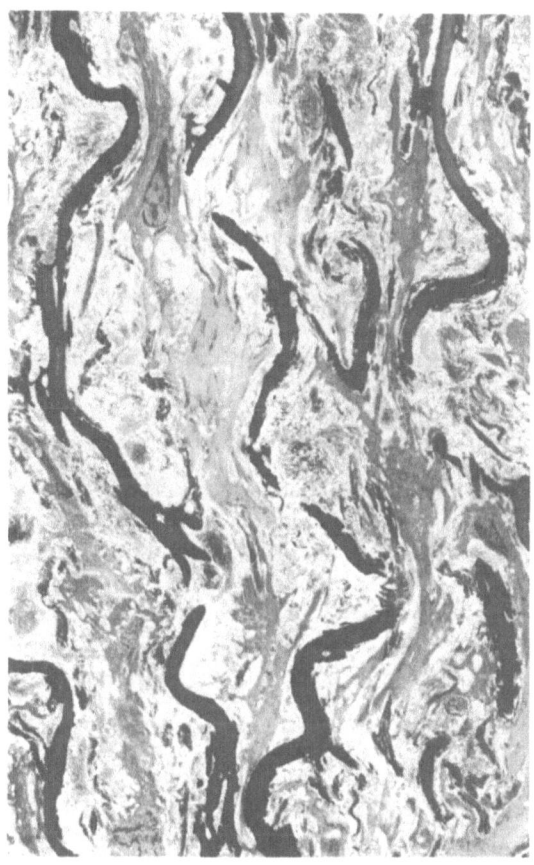

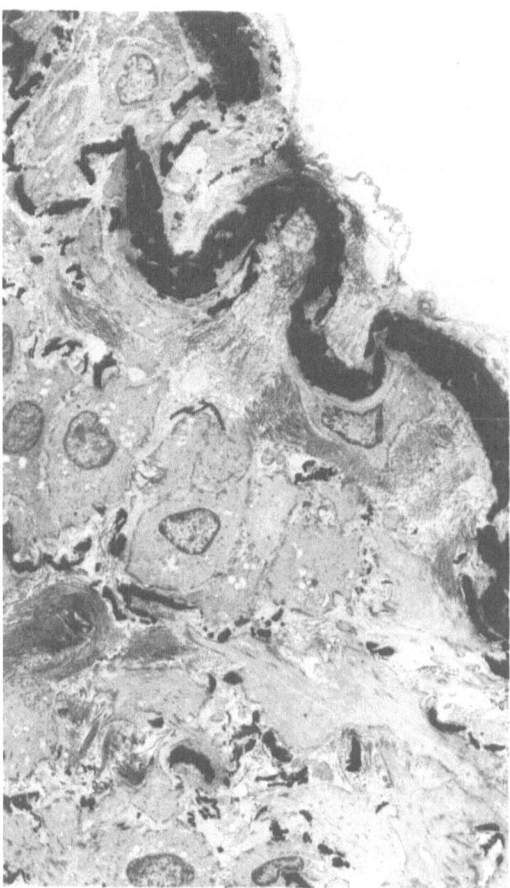

Fig. 5. Electron micrograph showing functional units of the media in an elastic type artery. There are more or less parallel elastic lamellae with smooth muscle cells, elastin fragments and collagen fibers sandwiched in between.

Fig. 6. Electron micrograph of the media of a muscular artery. Smooth muscle cells are closely packed with sparse elastin and collagen fibers in between. The internal elastic lamina stains densely (right upper corner).

echographic pictures may correlate well with gross and histological assessments of these parameters. At that stage, however, the gain of ultrasound imaging within the clinical setting may be questionable.

Detection of early atherosclerotic lesions creates a problem, mainly because of uncertainties with respect to the interpretation of intimal thickening once visualized. Thickening of the intima does not necessarily indicate an atherosclerotic lesion. Diffuse intimal thickening, for instance, occurs almost as a natural phenomenon and should not necessarily be considered as a 'precursor' lesion for atherosclerosis. Within diffuse intimal thickening areas may occur with a cellular immune response, alike that encountered in well defined atherosclerotic

lesions, but these observations cannot be generalized. Indeed, it is more likely that diffuse intimal thickening itself should be considered 'fertile soil' for atherogenesis, rather than a pertinent precursor lesion. Having said this, a major problem has risen for the investigator using ultrasound imaging techniques. How to differentiate between a 'natural' phenomenon (despite the fact that we do not know whether it is strictly speaking a pathological or physiological phenomenon) and lesions which are truly early atherogenetic? This problem is real, particularly, since in early atherogenesis pooling of lipids is not yet the case.

The restrictions eluded to above should then be

considered also in the light of differences in tissue characteristics of the arteries studied. A muscular media appears to be hypoechoic, while the media of an elastic type artery is highly echogenic. The latter thus interferes with an adequate visualization of the intima. To complicate matters further many arterial segments are transitional between 'truly' muscular and elastic.

Hence, it may well be that further technological developments are necessary in order to be able to distinguish between the 'real' atherogenetic early lesion and changes which will not by necessity progress to be full blown picture. This then is of major clinical impact and, for the time being, sets the limitations for the clinical application of this intravascular technique.

References

1. Becker AE. Atherosclerosis – a lesion in search of a definition. Int J Cardiol 1985; 8: 375–7.
2. McBride W, Lange RA, Hillis LD. Restenosis after successful coronary angioplasty. Pathophysiology and prevention. N Engl J Med 1988; 318: 1734–7.
3. Ross R. The pathogenesis of atherosclerosis – an update. N Engl J Med 1986; 314: 488–500.
4. Wal AC van der, Das PK, Bentz van de Berg D, Loos CM, Becker AE. Atherosclerotic lesions in man. In situ immunophenotypic analysis suggesting an immune mediated response. Lab Invest 1989 (in press).
5. Gown AM, Tsukada T, Ross R. Human atherosclerosis II. Immunocytochemical analysis of the cellular composition of human atherosclerotic lesions. Am J Pathol 1986; 125: 191–207.
6. Gussenhoven WJ, Essed CE, Lancée CT, Mastik F, Frietman P, Egmond FC van, Reiber J, Bosch H, Urk H van, Roelandt J, Bom N. Intravascular echographic assessment of vessel wall characteristics: a correlation with histology. Int J Cardiac Imaging 1989; 4: 105–116.

International Journal of Cardiac Imaging **4**: 105–116, 1989.
© 1989 *Kluwer Academic Publishers.*

Intravascular echographic assessment of vessel wall characteristics: a correlation with histology

W.J. Gussenhoven[1,5], C.E. Essed[2]*, P. Frietman[1], F. Mastik[1], C. Lancée[1], C. Slager[1], P. Serruys[1], P. Gerritsen[3], H. Pieterman[4] & N. Bom[1]
Academic Hospital Dijkzigt and Erasmus University, Departments of [1]Thoraxcenter, [2] Clinical Pathology, [3] Vascular Surgery, [4] Radiology and [5] The Interuniversity Cardiology Institute of the Netherlands

Summary

In vivo application of intravascular high frequency ultrasonic imaging for peripheral and coronary artery disease is a promising technique for vascular surgeons, radiologists and cardiologists. This report demonstrates in vitro results obtained with a high frequency imaging catheter (40 MHz) in 70 human specimens including arteries with and without atherosclerosis, veins, coronary artery bypass grafts and vascular prosthetic material. Correlation between the ultrasonic images and the histologic characteristics of the corresponding vessel wall tissue and lumen geometry was established. In addition, the effect of intervention techniques i.e. balloon angioplasty, spark erosion and laser were studied with ultrasound and histology. It is anticipated that development of such a catheter imaging technique has potential for diagnostic imaging and for combination with therapeutic systems.

Introduction

The ultimate advantage of intravascular ultrasonic catheters is that its unique position allows the use of high frequency transducers (> 20 MHz) which provide detailed information of both vessel geometry and morphology.

The ability of intravascular ultrasound to assess in vitro the diameter, area and wall thickness of the artery and to distinguish calcified from non-calcified atherosclerotic lesions has been reported [1–5]. Our own experience revealed the possibility to distinguish muscular from elastic arteries as well as to differentiate between the basic components of atherosclerosis [6–7].

This report has two principle aims. First, to acquaint future intravascular ultrasonographers with the **histologic** characteristics of arteries, veins, aorta-coronary artery bypass grafts, vascular prostheses and atherosclerosis. Subsequently, these data are compared with the **ultrasonic** characteristics obtained in a series of in vitro studies using human vascular specimens.

Second, the basic aspects of intervention techniques i.e. balloon dilatation, spark erosion and laser are outlined. Subsequently, the effect of these intervention techniques as visualized by ultrasound using human vascular specimens are evaluated. The results are compared with those from the corresponding histologic sections.

Technique

All studies were performed with a high frequency intravascular device currently under development at our laboratory. A 40 MHz single element transducer mounted on a 8F catheter tip was used. Axial

---

* Dr. C.E. Essed is presently working at the laboratory of Volksgezondheid in Friesland, Leeuwarden, The Netherlands.

resolution of the system was 75 μm. Lateral resolution was better than 200 μm at a depth of 1 mm. Cross-sectional images were obtained by motor-driven catheter tip rotation. Data acquisition time to complete one image was 20 seconds. The resulting images were displayed on a monitor via a video scanned memory.

Human specimens

Specimens were either removed at surgery or at autopsy. The specimens of approximately 10 mm length were isolated from redundant surrounding tissues and were stored at $-20°$C. For in vitro studies a total of 70 specimens were selected; arteries (54) (common carotid, subclavian, internal thoracic, brachial, coronary, superior mesenteric, splenic, renal, iliac and femoral); veins (4) (splenic, iliac, femoral, and saphenous); aorta-coronary bypass grafts (4) and segments of vascular prosthetic material (Goretex; Stent) (8). Atherosclerotic lesions were present to a variable degree.

For in vitro studies the specimens were thawed and embedded in a 1.2% solution of agar-agar. The specimens were positioned vertically in order to allow adequate access of the ultrasound catheter. The lumen of the specimens was filled with purified water.

In vitro experiments were carried out by placing the catheter in the lumen of the specimen. Subsequently, ultrasonic cross-sections were obtained from proximal to distal with 1 mm interval between each.

Microscopic investigation

The proximal cross-sectional sites of the specimens were correspondingly marked with ink. Subsequently they were fixed in 10% buffered formalin, decalcified and processed for routine paraffin embedding. Transverse sections of 5 μm thick perpendicular to the longitudinal axis of the vessel were cut at 1 mm intervals. The sections, arranged from proximal to distal, were stained with a Verhoeff's elastin van Gieson and the Haematoxylin azophloxine technique [8].

Data analysis

From each of the 70 specimens studied the characteristics, as documented by histology, were compared with the corresponding echo cross-section.

Results

Arteries

Histology
Basically there are 2 types of arteries – elastic and muscular [9]. The 2 types are not sharply divided since elastic arteries gradually merge into muscular arteries.

The aorta, pulmonary trunk and its main branches, and the proximal segments of the brachiocephalic, carotid, subclavian and common iliac arteries belong to the elastic type. All other arteries such as the coronary, renal and femoral, are muscular.

Histologically, the wall of both types of artery is composed of an intima, an internal elastic lamina, a media, an external elastic lamina and an adventitia. The main difference between the 2 types of arteries is found in the composition of the media.

In the elastic artery the media consists of circularly arranged elastin fibers which have smooth muscle cells sandwiched in between (Fig. 1). This makes the media of this type of artery elastin-rich. There may be a varying amount of intercellular connective tissue and mucopolysaccharide-rich ground substance. In the muscular artery the media predominantly consists of circularly arranged smooth muscle cells (Fig. 1). Only a few elastin fibers may be present, particularly within the larger arteries, as well as some intercellular connective tissue.

Echography
Based on the typical histologic differences found in the composition of the media, accurate distinction was possible between the different types of arteries studied. An elastic artery was recognized by a media which was as echogenic as the surrounding intima and adventitia. The presence of circularly

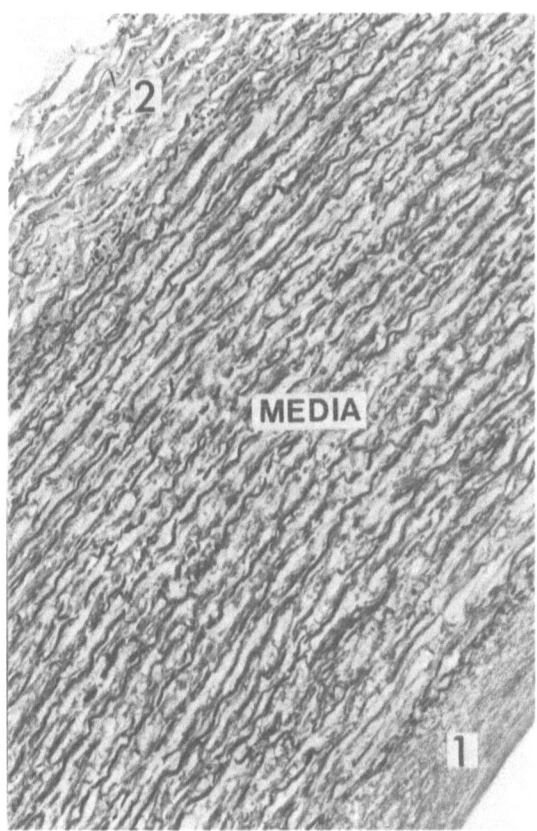 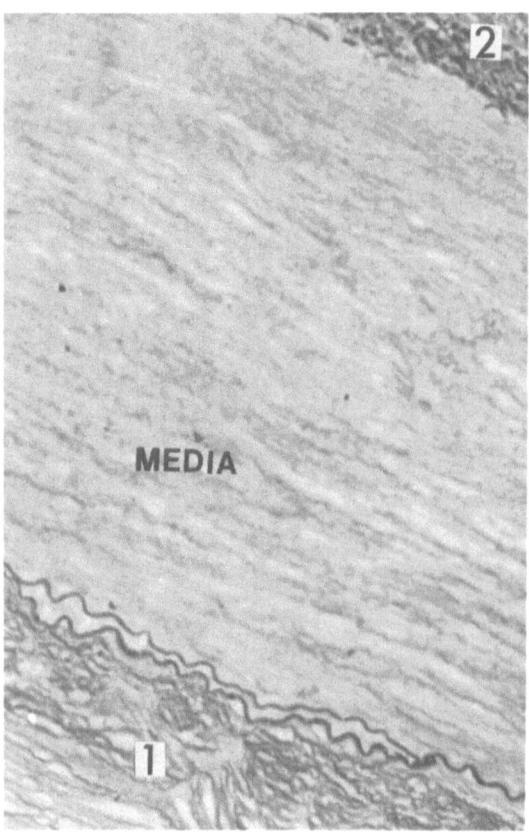

Fig. 1. Photomicrographs showing detailed characteristics of the media of an elastic artery (left panel) and a muscular artery (right panel) interposed between intima (1) and adventitia (2). The media of an elastic artery is densely packed with elastin fibers (black stained) whereas the media of a muscular artery is mainly composed of smooth muscle cells. Verhoeff van Gieson stain. Original magnification 60x.

arranged elastin fibers in the media of an elastic artery resulted in a significant amount of acoustic backscatter with a power level comparable to that from the surrounding tissues (Fig. 2).

Conversely, muscular arteries presented as a typical three-layered wall: an hypoechoic media amidst the intima and adventitia, both showing bright echoes (Figs. 2, 3).

Based on the ultrasonic appearance of the media (bright or hypoechoic) intravascular ultrasound provided a correct distinction between elastic (22) and muscular arteries (32). The aorta, carotid, subclavian and internal thoracic arteries presented as elastic arteries (Fig. 2). The brachial, coronary, mesenteric, splenic, renal, iliac (distal) and femoral arteries were of a muscular nature (Figs. 2, 3).

With ultrasound we were able to observe that an elastic artery gradually merges into a muscular artery based on the echo characteristics of the media. Studies in proximal coronary artery specimens revealed that the media of the artery was of an elastic nature, whereas 2–3 mm distally the media became progressively more muscular (Fig. 2).

In our experience both the intima and internal elastic lamina and the external elastic lamina and adventitia could not be discriminated by ultrasound.

Veins

Histology

Veins have thinner walls than their arterial companion. They contain an abundance of connective

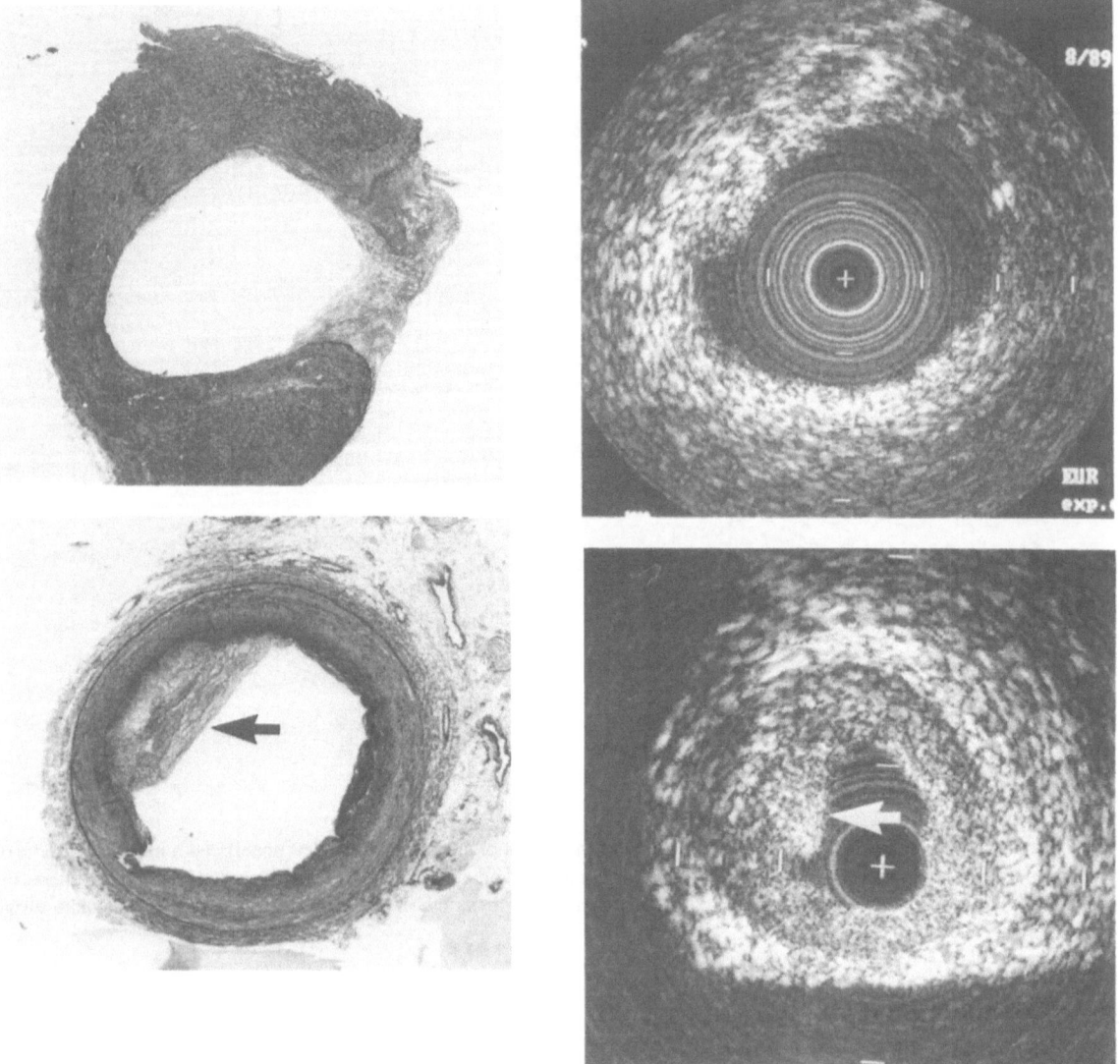

Fig. 2. Photomicrographs showing the difference in architecture of the media in the proximal left main coronary artery. At the junction of the aortic root the media is of elastin nature (upper panel). It consists of densely-packed multi-layered elastin fibers, an observation much facilitated by utilizing a selective elastin staining technique. On the corresponding ultrasonic cross-section the media appears to be as bright as the intima and adventitia.

The section obtained 2 mm distally (lower panel) shows the media to be of muscular nature. It is mainly composed of smooth muscle cells whereas the elastin fibers are more or less disorganized. The media on the corresponding ultrasonic cross-section appears relatively hypoechoic. An eccentric atherosclerotic lesion, best seen between 9 and 12 o'clock in the lower panel, is composed of fibromuscular tissue and lipid (arrow). On ultrasound the lesion (arrow) was recognized by soft echoes with bright particles. Verhoeff van Gieson stain. Magnification 8x.

tissue, whereas elastin fibers and smooth muscle cells occur in smaller numbers. Consequently their lumen is often collapsed during routine preparation for light microscopy.

The structure of small and **medium** sized veins varies greatly. Histologically, the wall consists of basically 3 unclearly defined layers: intima, media and adventitia. The intima consists of endothelial cells which either rest directly on a poorly defined internal elastic lamina or are separated from it by a

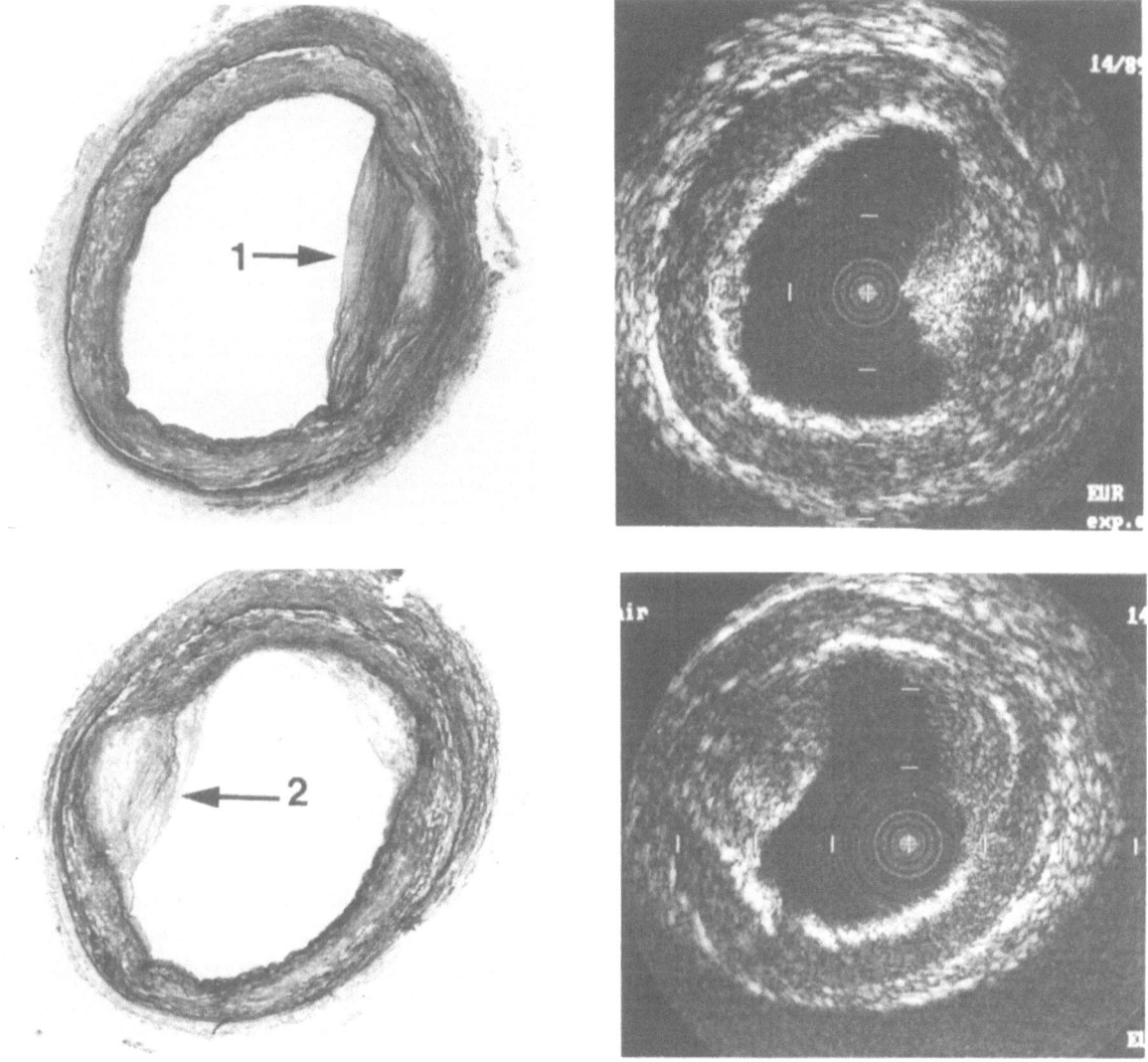

Fig. 3. Photomicrographs of histologic cross-sections obtained from the mesenteric superior artery together with the corresponding ultrasonic cross-sections. The media of this typical muscular artery mainly composed of smooth muscle cells, appears characteristically hypoechoic on ultrasound. Note that the eccentric atherosclerotic lesion barely visible at 9 o'clock (upper panel) is of marked larger size compared to the cross-section obtained 4 mm distally (lower panel). Both lesions (arrows 1 and 2) were of amorphous non-calcific tissue character containing fibromuscular tissue and lipid. Bright echoes of intima and adventitia circumscribing the hypoechoic media. Verhoeff van Gieson stain. Magnification 8x.

slight amount of subendothelial connective tissue. The media consists of circularly, or circularly and longitudinally, disposed smooth muscle cells and collagen, and few elastin fibers. The external elastic lamina is poorly defined. The adventitia consists mainly of thick collagen-rich connective tissue arranged longitudinally. It is the thickest part of the wall blending with the media [9].

Echography

Compared to the ultrasonic gain setting necessary to image arterial wall specimens, a higher gain setting was required to get a proper image of the veins. The walls of the veins studied produced soft echoes which did not allow any ultrasonic distinction between intima, media and adventitia (Fig. 4). This is intimately related to the composition of the

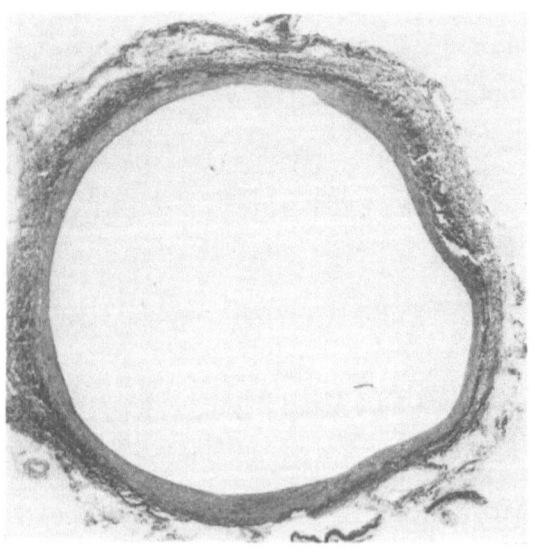 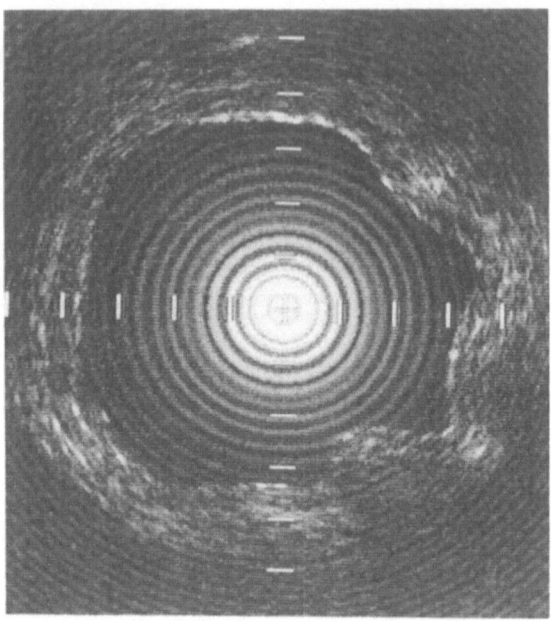

Fig. 4. Microphotograph of a histologic section and corresponding intravascular ultrasonic cross-section obtained from the femoral vein. Intima, media and adventitia cannot be distinguished with ultrasound. Verhoeff van Gieson stain. Magnification 8x.

wall: predominantly composed of fibrous connective tissue and smooth muscle cells. Whereas elastin fibers, commonly present in the internal and external elastic lamina, were practically absent.

Aorta-coronary artery bypass grafts

Histology

Following aorta-coronary bypass grafting the autologous saphenous vein, used in this procedure, may show adaptive and reparative changes [10]. These are superimposed upon any preexisting changes in the vein. Damage to endothelial cells in the early phase after grafting leads to fibrin deposits on the intimal surface and edema of the wall. After 4–6 weeks proliferation of myointimal cells may cause intima thickening. Over years this may progress to classical atherosclerotic lesions [10].

The media is affected by interference with its blood supply caused by transplantation and the muscle cells may die and be replaced by connective or collagen-rich connective tissue (fibrosis). Remaining muscle cells may hypertrophy. The adventitia on the other hand becomes replaced by scarred and collagen-rich connective tissue (fibrosis).

Echography

The main ultrasonic changes that occurred in saphenous veins used for aorta-coronary artery bypass surgery were proliferation of myointimal cells recognized as a zone of soft echoes, and fibrosis of media and adventitia recognized as bright echoes (Fig. 5). Both latter structures could not be differentiated from each other with ultrasound, as was the case with normal veins.

Vascular prostheses

Histology

The synthetic Goretex material appeared on histology as well-arranged, short-fiber elements. For obvious reasons stents are not amenable to be sectioned histologically. In the early postoperative phase the lumen surface of a vascular prosthesis becomes covered by fibrin deposits; later to be replaced by fibromuscular tissue.

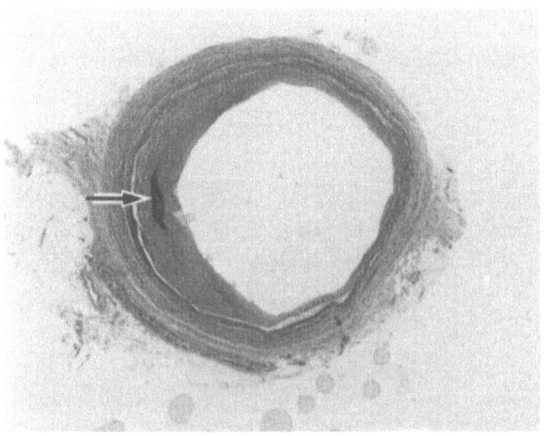 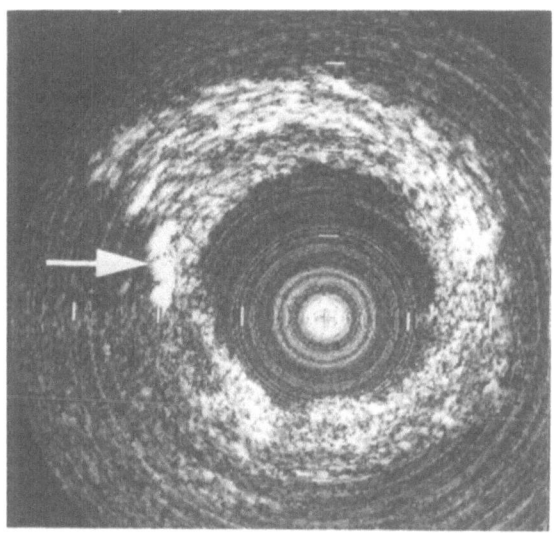

Fig. 5. Photomicrograph showing the architecture of an implanted venous bypass graft and corresponding ultrasonic cross-section. Histologically, the adventitia is composed of collagen-rich connective tissue and the media shows diffuse fibrosis. Between 6 and 12 o'clock a superimposed atherosclerotic lesion is seen which mainly consists of connective tissue with diffuse lipid deposits. On ultrasound a more echoreflective zone is seen between 11 and 3 o'clock reflective of scarred adventitial tissue. The scarred adventitia between 3 and 11 o'clock is not detected with ultrasound presumably due to an inappropriate angle of the ultrasound beam in respect to the adventitia. The atherosclerotic lesion appears with soft echoes. Calcium present at 9 o'clock (arrow) causes ultrasonic shadowing. Haematoxylin azophloxine stain. Magnification 8x.

Echography

On ultrasound the Goretex prosthesis as well as the stent were recognized as a highly reflective, relatively thin structure. Fibrin deposits as well as fibromuscular tissue were recognized as soft echoes (Fig. 6).

Atherosclerotic lesions

Histology

Early atherosclerotic lesions are known as fatty streaks and are composed of agglomerates of foam cells containing lipids. The advanced lesion, the atherosclerotic plaque, shows extensive variability in its composition. At one end of the spectrum the atherosclerotic plaque may be almost entirely composed of fibromuscular tissue i.e. connective tissue, smooth muscle cells and disorganized elastin fibers with an important collagenous component. At the other end, the plaque may consist of a large central atheroma with a scanty fibrous capsule composed of collagen-rich connective tissue.

The classical atherosclerotic plaque is localized in the intima and is composed of a lake of fatty debris with cholesterol crystals, sometimes fibrin and calcium deposits – the atheroma surrounded by macrophages and lymphocytes and a fibromuscular layer. Towards the lumen the lesion is bordered by a fibrous tissue capsule covered by endothelium. Towards the media the border of the plaque may be easily recognizable by a still present internal elastic lamina, but may also be vague due to the presence of a fibromuscular layer. In some instances the internal elastic lamina and the media may even totally disappear and the atherosclerotic lesion can reach as far as the adventitia. Such a lesion will evoke an inflammatory infiltrate in the adventitia [11]. When the fibrous capsule becomes extremely thin it may rupture and allow blood and blood components to enter the plaque leading to plaque haemorrhage.

A complication of a ruptured or cracked plaque is thrombus formation on its surface. The thrombus is composed of a meshwork of strands of fibrin in which red cells, leukocytes and platelets are en-

112

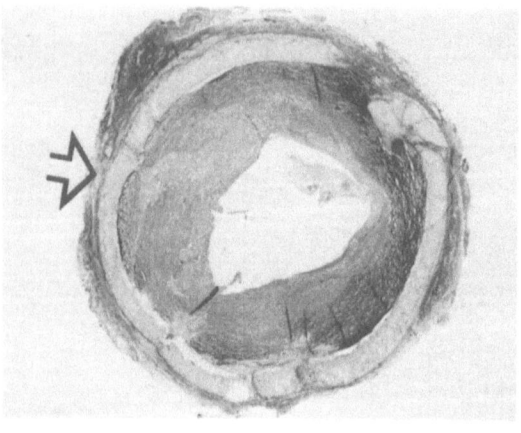
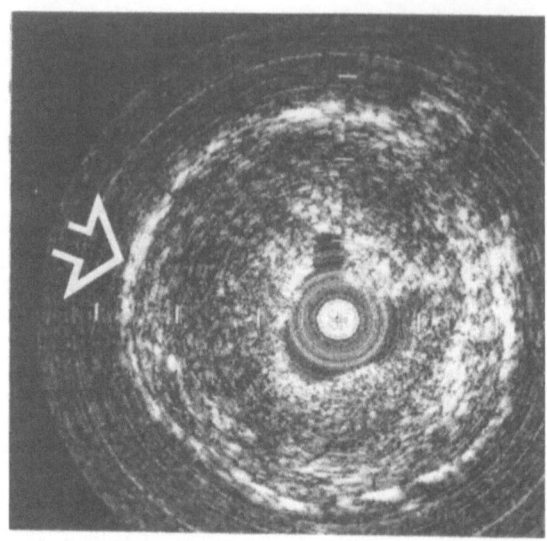

Fig. 6. Microphotograph showing a vascular Goretex prosthesis in cross-section with an obstructive lesion. The lesion consists mainly of loose connective tissue. On the corresponding ultrasound cross-section the Goretex prosthesis is recognized as a reflective structure (open arrow). The lesion itself generates relatively soft echoes. Verhoeff van Gieson stain. Magnification 8x.

trapped. If the thrombus does not dissolve it becomes organized by ingrowth of fibrovascular tissue [12].

Echography

Based on the echogenicity of the atherosclerotic lesion, ultrasound could distinguish 4 basic types of plaque components:

1. hypoechoic – a reflection of a significant deposit of lipid (Fig. 7).
2. soft echoes – reflective of fibromuscular tissue (intimal proliferation as well as lesions that consist of fibromuscular tissue and diffusely dispersed lipid: the atherosclerotic lesion, Figs. 2, 3, 5 and 8).
3. bright echoes – representative for collagen-rich fibrous tissues (Fig. 7).
4. bright echoes with shadowing behind the lesion, representative for calcium (Figs. 5 and 7).

Of the 54 arteries studied there was no histologic evidence of atherosclerosis in 4: this was confirmed with intravascular imaging. In 7 specimens fibromuscular tissue was the only underlying disorder and on ultrasound it was recognized as soft echoes adjacent to the intimal surface. In the remaining 43

arteries histology revealed the presence of an atherosclerotic lesion, either restricted to one particular area (19) or involving the entire arterial vessel circumference (24). Ultrasound examination had correctly assessed the presence and extent of the lesion involved. By systematically scanning the arteries with ultrasound from proximal to distal, at a 1 mm interval, it was noted that the location and composition of atherosclerotic plaques revealed marked variations (Figs. 3 and 7).

Interventional techniques in relation to intravascular echography

In a separate series of 16 human specimens with an obstructive atherosclerotic lesion the effect of balloon dilatation, spark erosion and laser on the tissue interrogated was assessed echographically and compared to histology.

Balloon dilatation

With help of a balloon catheter, obstructive lesions in both femoral and iliac arteries were dilated. For this purpose a Cordis 4F (femoral) and 7F (iliac)

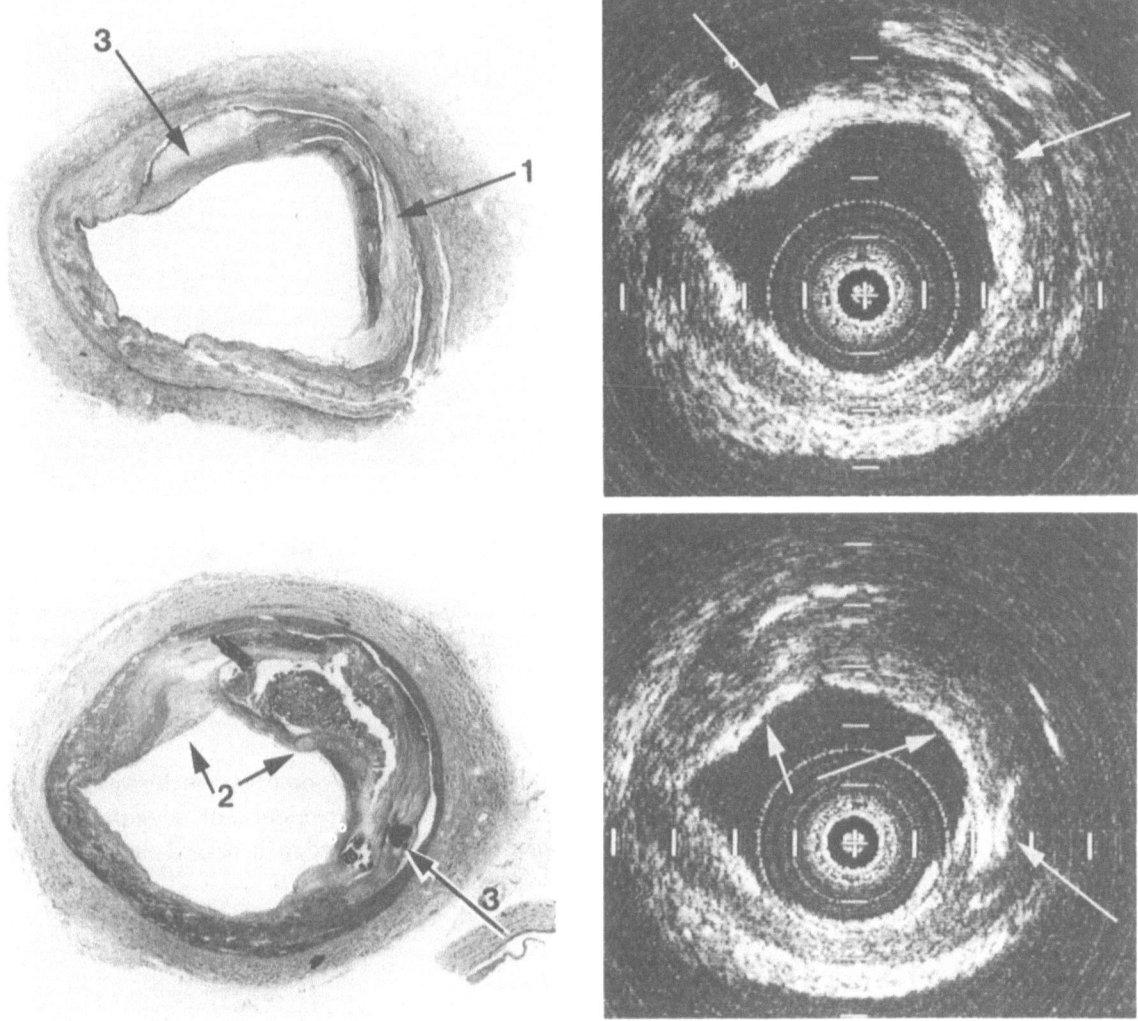

Fig. 7. Histologic cross-sections of a femoral artery showing a classical obstructive atherosclerotic lesion with corresponding ultrasonic cross-sections. Fatty debris appearing as hypoechoic (arrow 1), collagen as bright echoes (arrow 2) and calcium as bright echoes with shadowing (arrow 3), are the major plaque constituents. Distribution of calcium within the lesion varies significantly (11 o'clock in upper panel, 4 o'clock in lower panel). Verhoeff van Gieson stain upper panel. Haematoxylin azophloxin stain lower panel. Magnification 8x.

catheter were used and inflated to 10 Bar for one minute. Echographic investigation was performed before and 2 minutes following intervention. Care was taken to make the cross-sections, before and after the intervention, at comparable levels.

Histologically, a typical laceration of the plaque from the media was observed in all 4 specimens studied (Fig. 8). This observation is highly specific for a successful angioplastic procedure [13]. Ultrasound examination, however, revealed a distinct dissection in one of total 40 cross-sections studied, as an echo-free zone between the lesion and the original wall (Fig. 8). In 2 other cross-sections a dissection was questionable. It should be realized that these investigations were performed under non-physiologic conditions and might not be comparable to the situation in vivo. Therefore, it may be anticipated that after dilatation the dissected lesion remained adherent to the vessel wall. Furthermore, it was noted that the increase in lumen

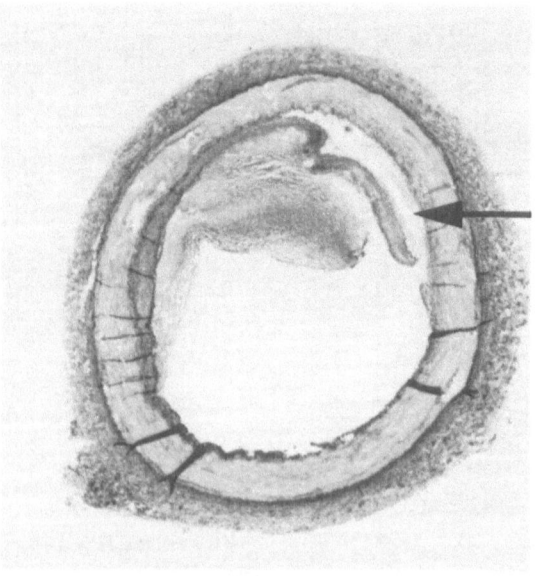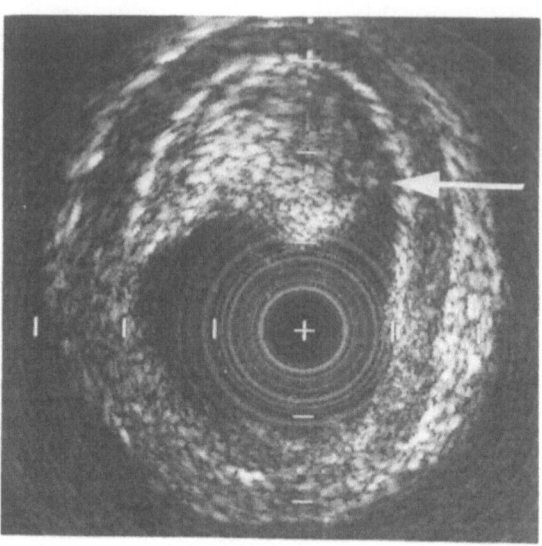

Fig. 8. Histologic and corresponding ultrasonic cross-sections obtained from the femoral artery after angioplasty. The artery presents an eccentric obstructive atherosclerotic lesion recognized as relatively soft echoes. The corresponding histologic cross-section shows that the lesion mainly consists of connective tissue and fatty deposits. The dilatation procedure had resulted in a dissection (arrow). Verhoeff van Gieson stain. Magnification 8x.

diameter after the procedure varied from no measurable increase to a lumen diameter increase twice its original size.

Spark erosion

Spark erosion was accomplished with a 2 mm diameter, parabolically shaped electrode which rotated at 750 rpm. The active electrode area used for spark erosion was 1 square mm. Sparking was applied during 40 ms periods at 1 sec intervals by application of 500 kHz alternating voltage with an effective value of 360 Volt [14].

This procedure was performed in 8 human arteries. In 6 of these arteries the lumen was totally occluded by an atherosclerotic lesion. For this reason spark erosion was performed in order to create an access for the ultrasonic transducer. One hour following the intervention the arteries were systematically studied with ultrasound. The presence of a distinct hole could be precisely identified and its location was subsequently confirmed by histology (Fig. 9). In all instances erosion of the plaque

surface was seen. Some of the histologic cross-sections revealed evidence of coagulation. This phenomenon resulted in increased ultrasonic back-scatter.

Laser

A 1.8 mm diameter rounded sapphire contact probe mounted on a 0.6 mm core silica fiber was used. The silica fiber was connected to a continuous wave Nd-YAG laser (Medilas-2, MBB). A saline flush (3 ml/min) prevented blood from entering the fiber-sapphire interface and cooled the sapphire crystal and the metal connector [15, 16]. Laser shots of 14 Watt power and exposure time of 20–40 seconds duration were used in 4 arteries, with lumens that were totally occluded by atherosclerotic lesions. This was done in order to create a lumen accessible for the ultrasound probe. Similar to the spark erosion technique, laser caused erosion of the plaque surface as well as some coagulation effect. The amount of coagulation was, in our experience, too minute to be detectable with ultrasound.

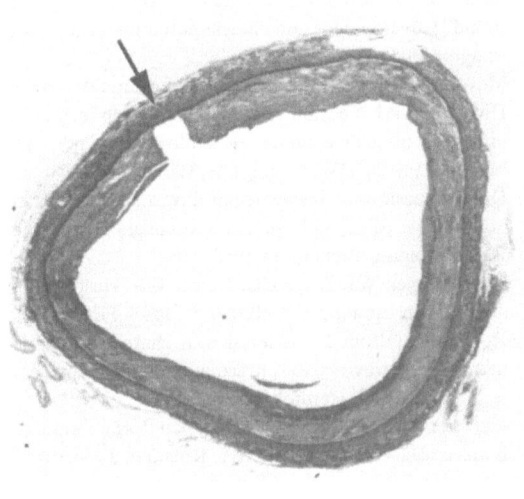
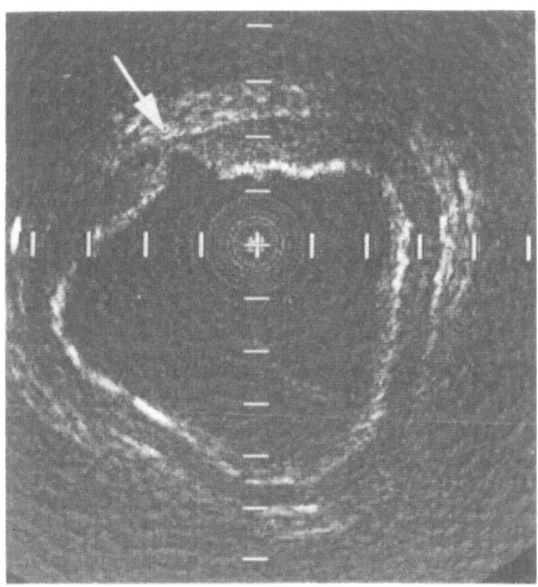

Fig. 9. Histologic and corresponding ultrasonic cross-section obtained from the iliac artery after spark erosion. At 11 o'clock a distinct hole is seen (arrow) created by spark erosion. Verhoeff van Gieson stain. Magnification 8x.

Limitations

The ultimate ultrasonic response is intimately dependent on the angle of insonification. Perpendicular insonification results in an optimal response (see also Figs. 2, 3 and 5). Only under these conditions are we able to make adequate distinction between the size and composition of the atherosclerotic lesion involved. This observation should be taken into account when in vivo application is considered.

Identification of atherosclerotic lesions in a muscular artery in general is facilitated by the presence of a highly reflective intima and a hypoechoic media. Conversely, adequate discrimination of the lesion from the underlying elastic artery may be prevented when the echo characteristics of the lesion are similar to the echo response generated by the intima and media in these elastic arteries (see also Fig. 2).

Conclusions

This report briefly reviews the histologic characteristics of human vascular specimens. The relation-ship between histology and cross-sectional ultrasonic images obtained with a high frequency transducer was studied in vitro.

A clear difference between elastin and muscular arteries was observed with ultrasound which was caused by the presence or absence of elastin tissue in the media. Moreover, the technique revealed characteristic differences in architecture of normal veins and veins used for aortacoronary bypass grafting. Vascular prostheses have a distinct influence on ultrasound as has its internal lumen surface.

Comparison between ultrasonic images and corresponding histologic cross-sections showed that characteristics of the echo image of an atherosclerotic lesion relate to the histologic composition of the lesion.

The effect of intervention techniques was studied. A typical plaque rupture following balloon dilatation may be observed. Spark erosion as well as laser intervention may produce coagulation which might result in an area of increased echoreflectivity.

This unique high resolution ultrasonic imaging device enables determination of the vessel and plaque morphology as well as assessment of the

116

extent of the disease. Application of such a technique is two-fold. First, for diagnostic imaging, the lumen area as well as characteristics of the type of lesion can be depicted. Knowledge of the plaque type enables prediction of the intervention procedure of choice and potential areas of difficulty. If the plaque is mainly non-calcific the lesion can be treated more easily than the calcified plaque. Second, the technique can be used as a control system after an intervention.

Acknowledgement

Our appreciation is extended to International Medical Zutphen, The Netherlands, who kindly enabled secretarial support for this manuscript. We thank Esther Clarke for providing tissue specimens, Coby Peekstok for preparing the histologic sections, Willem van Alphen and Leo Bekkering who constructed the transducer and colleagues of the department of Professor Dr. P. Verdouw for their consistent support.

Product Centre TNO and TPD-TNO Delft are acknowledged for their support to the design of the catheter prototype.

Supported by the Interuniversity Cardiology Institute of The Netherlands, The Netherlands Technology Foundation (STW) under grant number RGN.77.1257, the Dutch Ministry of Economic Affairs and The Netherlands Heart Foundation.

References

1. Pandian NG, Kreis A, Brockway B, Isner JM, Sacharoff A, Boleza E, Caro R, Muller D. Ultrasound angioscopy: Real-time, two-dimensional, intraluminal ultrasound imaging of blood vessels. Am J Cardiol 1988; 62: 493–4.
2. Linker DT, Yock PG, Thapliyal HV et al. *In vitro* analysis of backscattered amplitude from normal and diseased arteries using a new intraluminal ultrasonic catheter. JACC 1988; 11: 4A.
3. Yock PG, Johnson EL, Linker DT. Intravascular ultrasound. Development and clinical potential. Am J Cardiac Imaging 1988; 2: 185–93.
4. Meyer CR, Chiang BS, Fechner KP, Fitting DW, Williams DM, Buda AJ. Feasibility of high resolution intravascular ultrasonic imaging catheters. Radiology 1988; 168: 113–6.
5. Meyer S, Fitting DW, Chiang EH, Williams DM, Buda AJ. Development of an intravascular ultrasonic catheter imaging system. SPIE Vol. 904. Microsensors and Catheter-Based Imaging Technology 1988: 116–7.
6. Gussenhoven WJ, Essed CE, Lancée CT, Mastik F, Frietman P, van Egmond FC, Reiber J, Bosch H, van Urk H, Roelandt J, Bom N. Arterial wall characteristics determined by intravascular ultrasound imaging: an *in vitro* study. J Am Coll Cardiol (in press).
7. Gussenhoven WJ, Essed CE, Frietman P, van Egmond FC, Lancée CT, van Cappellen WA, Roelandt J, Serruys PW, Gerritsen GP, van Urk H, Bom N. Intravascular ultrasonic imaging: histologic and echographic correlation. Eur J Vasc Surg (in press).
8. Lillie RD, Fullmer HM. Connective tissue fibers and membranes. In: Histopathologic technique and practical histochemistry. London: McGraw-Hill Company, 1976: 679–718.
9. Ham AW. Histology. Chapter 22: The circulatory system. Oxford: Blackwell Scientific Publications, 1969: 581–691.
10. Silver MD, Wilson GJ. Pathology of cardiovascular prostheses including coronary artery bypass and other vascular grafts. In: Silver MD, ed. Cardiovascular pathology, Vol II. New York: Churchill Livingstone, 1983: 1225–96.
11. Haust MD. Atherosclerosis – lesions and sequelae. In: Silver MD, ed. Cardiovascular pathology, Vol II. New York: Churchill Livingstone, 1983: 191–315.
12. Anderson JR. Disturbances of blood flow and body fluids. In: Anderson JR, ed. Muir's textbook of pathology. London: Edward Arnold, 1985: 10.1–10.47.
13. Essed CE, van den Brand M, Becker AE. Transluminal coronary angioplasty and early stenosis. Fibrocellular occlusion after wall laceration. Br Heart J 1983; 49: 393–6.
14. Slager CJ, Essed CE, Schuurbiers JCH, Bom N, Serruys PW, Meester GT. Vaporization of atherosclerotic plaques by spark erosion. J Am Coll Cardiol 1985; 5: 1382–6.
15. Geschwind HJ, Blair JD, Monkolsmai D et al. Development and experimental application of contact probe catheter for laser angioplasty. J Am Coll Cardiol 1987; 9: 101–7.
16. Verdaasdonk RM, Cross FW, Borst C. Physical properties of sapphire fibre tips for laser angioplasty. Lasers Med Sci 1987; 2: 183–8.

International Journal of Cardiac Imaging **4**: 117–125, 1989.
© 1989 *Kluwer Academic Publishers.*

Clinical applications of intravascular ultrasound imaging in atherectomy

Paul G. Yock, David T. Linker[1], Neal W. White, Michael H. Rowe[2], Matthew R. Selmon[2], Gregory C. Robertson[2], Tomoaki Hinohara[2] & John B. Simpson[2]
Cardiovascular Research Institute and Division of Cardiology, M-1186 University of California, San Francisco, CA 94127, USA; [1]*Department of Biomedical Engineering and Division of Cardiology, University of Trondheim, N-7006 Trondheim, Norway;* [2]*Cardiac Catheterization Laboratory, Sequoia Hospital, Redwood City, California, USA*

Abstract

This paper discusses the potential application of intravascular ultrasound imaging in the context of catheter-based atherectomy. The advantages and limitations of ultrasound in this application are discussed, and representative cases are presented.

Introduction

Atherectomy is emerging as a major new therapeutic modality in the treatment of atherosclerotic vascular disease in both the peripheral and coronary arteries. Early experience with the various atherectomy catheters suggests that plaque extraction produces a more predictable result than balloon angioplasty, with a lower incidence of acute complications such as abrupt reclosure [1, 2]. In addition, it appears that the rates of restenosis may be lower than with balloon angioplasty [3]. The importance of this finding, if confirmed, is major: the ability to achieve substantially lower restenosis rates would undoubtedly cause a shift from balloon angioplasty to atherectomy as the procedure of choice for catheter treatment of atherosclerosis.

As experience with atherectomy is accumulating, it is becoming increasingly clear that imaging guidance provided by conventional angiography may not be sufficiently precise to guarantee maximally safe and effective procedures. It appears that restenosis rates can be minimized by aggressive removal of atheroma; however, this strategy increases the risk of vessel perforation. Intravascular ultrasound is ideally suited as a guidance modality

for atherectomy in this respect, since it is able to show the thickness of the vessel wall and the distribution of atheroma at any given level.

The purpose of this paper is to provide an overview of the potential application of intravascular ultrasound imaging in the context of atherectomy. The first section will describe the general types of atherectomy devices and discuss the initial clinical results being generated; in the second section, the potential utility of intravascular ultrasound imaging will be explored and compared with fiberoptic angioscopy; the third section will present some initial clinical results of imaging in the context of atherectomy; and a final section will outline some of the potential areas for further development in this area.

The atherectomy devices: Initial clinical studies

Terminology

The term 'atherectomy' was coined by Simpson to describe a catheter-based procedure in which atheroma is extracted in the form of intact specimens [1]. The term appears to be undergoing generalization, however, and will likely be used to describe any mechanical means of cutting or abrading plaque, whether or not the specimens are retrieved.

Basic designs

The atherectomy devices currently under development and testing can be broadly grouped into two categories. 'Directional' devices, of which the Simpson Atherocath (TM) is the prototype, extract plaque by cutting at one side of the catheter tip (see Fig. 1). These are debulking devices, with which an existing lumen is enlarged by virtue of removal of atheroma in selected portions of the circumference of the vessel. Because of this configuration, the ultimate lumen dimension generally exceeds the size of the catheter following a successful procedure. The coaxial devices cut in a generally forward fashion, either tunneling without guidance (the Kensey catheter [4]), or following a guidewire that is placed through a region of stenosis (the Auth Rotablator (TM) [5] and the transluminal extraction catheter (TEC, TM [6]). The coaxial devices enlarge the lumen in a symmetrical fashion, creating a new lumen which is equal in size to the diameter of the cutting element.

The devices also differ with respect to the mechanism of plaque removal. With the Simpson catheter, the plaque is shaved by a cutter which traps the material in a housing. After multiple passes with the cutter, the housing becomes filled and the catheter is removed for emptying. The TEC device is operated with suction applied to the proximal end of the catheter. The atheroma is broken into small pieces by the action of rotating blades at the tip of the catheter, and the pieces are drawn through the catheter by the suction and deposited in a collection chamber outside the body. The Rotablator and Kensey catheters allow the debris generated from the abrading and pulverizing action of the catheters to pass downstream. Since the bulk of the particulate material is less than 10 microns in diameter, the expectation is that there will not be clinically significant embolization to the distal vessels.

Initial clinical experience

Among the various catheters the Simpson atherectomy device has undergone the most extensive clinical testing to date. Peripheral trials have demonstrated primary success rates (reduction of stenosis to under 50%) ranging between 87 and 97% [1, 7]. Overall rates of restenosis average 31% at six months, with the most important predictor of restenosis being a post-procedure stenosis of greater than 30% as judged by angiography [3]. The incidence of perforation associated with the atherectomy device has been reported to be as high as 6.5% by Dorros and colleagues; their series, however, included total obstructions requiring the device to be forced through a lesion without clear visualization [7]. Simpson and colleagues have encountered no atherectomy-associated perforations in the peripheral vessels. Media has been seen histologically in approximately 5–10% of specimens removed; adventitia is sampled only rarely [8].

Initial reports of the results of coronary atherectomy with the Simpson device have also been encouraging. Following an initial learning period, the primary success rate reported by Simpson and colleagues at Sequoia Hospital was 90% [2]. One coronary artery perforation has occurred to date in this group's experience of over 200 procedures. Both media and adventitia are seen in the excised specimens in higher proportion than in the periphery, although the exact numbers are not yet tabulated [8]. One patient in whom adventitia was present in the biopsy specimen underwent repeat catheterization for angina, and was shown to have a significant aneurysm at the site of prior atherectomy. Data on restenosis following coronary atherectomy are still accumulating, although preliminary indications are that the restenosis rates may be as low as 18% in lesions not previously treated by angioplasty [9]. This contrasts with an average restenosis rate of 30–35% overall following balloon angioplasty.

Early clinical trials of the TEC catheter in peripheral vessels have also yielded high primary success rates (98% in the initial 41 procedures) [6]. No perforations or clinically significant distal embolization were encountered in these cases. Pilot trials

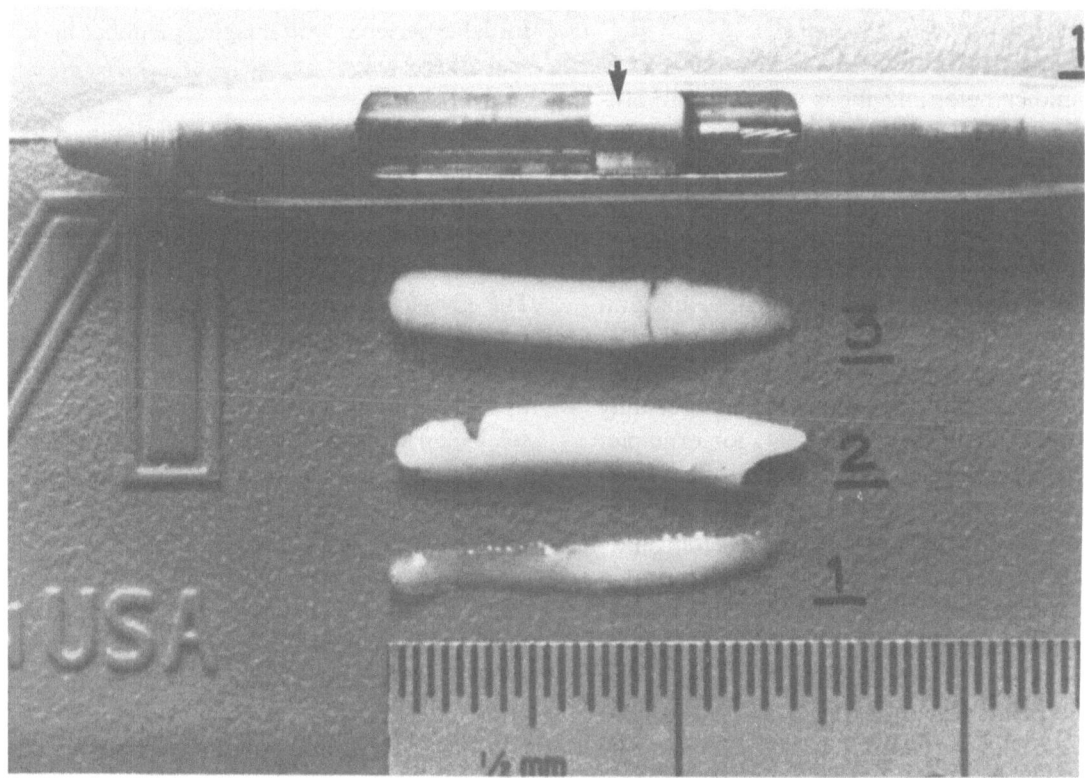

Fig. 1. Simpson atherectomy device shown with three atherectomy specimens. The open housing of the device faces outward in the photograph, revealing the cutter (arrow) which is connected to a rotating cable. Advancing the cutter shaves off a strip of atheroma, which is trapped in the forward portion of the housing (to the left in the figure).

of coronary endarterectomy have been performed recently with the Auth device in the context of bypass surgery [10] and via a standard percutaneous approach. The catheter has provided a smooth, regular lumen in most cases, although perforation and distal embolization have occurred.

The need for improved imaging

It is clear from the early experience with atherectomy that the technique can be performed with relatively high primary success rate. It also appears that the rates of restenosis may be significantly lower than for balloon angioplasty, depending on how completely atheroma is removed. Unfortunately, aggressive debulking of a vessel increases the risk of weakening the vessel wall (leading to subsequent aneurysm formation) or actually perforating the vessel acutely.

Angiography and angioscopy

Angiographic imaging techniques are unlikely to provide sufficiently accurate guidance to allow complete and careful excision of atheroma. Although a general idea of the distribution of plaque in the artery can be obtained from the contrast images, our experience suggests that the angiographic appearance is imprecise and often frankly misleading in identifying the thickness of plaque present in any given radial direction. High-resolution imaging with fiberoptic angioscopy has been applied in the context of atherectomy, but has principally been used to assess the smoothness of the atherectomy surface and to detect significant dissections [11]. Because the angioscope images only intimal and immediate subintimal tissues, it is unlikely to provide a useful guide for orienting a directional atherectomy device toward the thickest accumulation of atheroma.

Advantages of catheter ultrasound

Ultrasound catheter imaging is well suited to provide imaging guidance for atherectomy in several respects. Because detailed information about vessel wall composition can be obtained well below the intimal surface, the ultrasound images can be used to determine the most strategic positioning of cuts. Accurate information concerning plaque and vessel wall morphology may also be extremely useful in answering some significant practical questions which remain concerning the atherectomy procedure. It is unclear at present, for example, whether the entire thickness of an atheroma deposit should in fact be removed from the vessel wall: the media of diseased vessels can be significantly thinned and may not provide sufficient structural support for the vessel if all of the overlying atheroma is completely excised.

The image plane of the current ultrasound catheters – perpendicular to the catheter tip – is also favorable for the application to atherectomy. The operator can develop a detailed three-dimensional sense of the distribution of atheroma by moving the catheter axially back and forth through the region of interest. This information allows the operator to position the atherectomy device accurately with respect to axial position in the vessel, as well as directing the device radially to the appropriate segment of the wall.

The use of ultrasound imaging in the case of the coaxial atherectomy devices is also promising, although the application is different. Potentially, it may be very effective to scan a vessel once an initial, small-caliber channel is made in order to select the definitive catheter. Regions of highly eccentric atheroma deposition, particularly in portions of the vessel which bend or branch, may be less favorable for larger cutting diameters compared to straight vessel segments with concentric atheroma. Imaging may also help determine how far distally in a vessel it is safe to proceed with an imaging catheter of a given diameter.

Initial experience with imaging guidance in peripheral atherectomy

We have recently reported our preliminary experience using catheter ultrasound in the context of peripheral atherectomy [12]. The prototype ultrasound catheters were provided by Cardiovascular Imaging Systems, Inc. (Cvis) of Sunnyvale, CA. The Cvis catheters have a fixed crystal/rotating reflector mechanical transducer system which generates an image plane perpendicular to the catheter tip. The rotating reflector is shielded from the vessel by an acoustically transparent housing. The transducer frequency for the peripheral studies reported here was 20 MHz, providing a radial image penetration of approximately 1,5–2 cm. The catheters are guided by a fixed wire incorporated into the tip of the device. The wire can be shaped by the operator to help guide the catheter into the appropriate vessel or branch. Catheters are available in 5 and 8 French sizes; in general, the 8 French catheters have been used for the peripheral imaging studies because of the superior imaging characteristics provided by the larger transducer aperture. The catheters require filling with fluid before use in order to provide a bubble-free beam path from the transducer to the outside of the catheter. The Cvis imaging electronics (Ultrascan One (TM)) provide a real-time image of the vessel at frame rates between 15 and 30/second, depending on image depth.

Methods

Atherectomies were performed using the Simpson Atherocath (TM). In the pilot series of studies, the timing and frequency of ultrasound imaging during the procedure was at the discretion of the atherectomy operator. In general, imaging was not attempted prior to any intervention due to the operators' desire to begin the procedure with the atherectomy device. Imaging was usually performed at intervals during and at the completion of the case. In some patients, imaging was not attempted until the end of the procedure, when the angiographic results were felt to be satisfactory.

The logistics of introducing a separate imaging catheter were relatively straightforward. We found that the most efficient time for imaging was during a natural pause in the procedure during which the collection chamber of the atherectomy device is unloaded. This occurs at least several times during a typical peripheral case: although multiple cuts can be made during one passage of the atherectomy catheter, the amount of material removed is sufficient to fill the collecting chamber a number of times. This alternating sequence of cutting and imaging is a useful one, because it allows the operators to periodically identify regions of the vessel which require further work. We found that guiding the device to the appropriate vessel was not a problem in the periphery using the fixed guidewire system.

The major technical difficulty encountered in imaging involved initial filling of the catheters. The presence of even a small bubble caused significant deterioration in image quality. Successful filling of the prototype catheters typically required one to three minutes and was a function of experience with the filling procedure.

Orienting of the ultrasound image with respect to the patient position and the fluoroscopic images is an essential and nontrivial step. In the Cvis system, the catheters are provided with a narrow 'bridge' on one side of the acoustic housing which is visible both on fluoroscopy and on the ultrasound image. In order to correlate the image orientation with fluoroscopic position, the catheter is introduced into the vessel then rotated until the strut is at an identifiable position on the fluoroscopic image. We have found it easiest in practice to position the bridge laterally. The ultrasound image is then electronically rotated until the bridge indicator appears at the appropriate position on the screen – for example, at 3 o'clock. When this is accomplished, the image is oriented with respect to fluoroscopy and to the patient (up on the image is anterior, and so on). This orientation procedure is essential if the directional atherectomy device is to be positioned for cutting based on the ultrasound catheter images. The rotational position of the Simpson atherectomy catheter can also be determined fluoroscopically, so that the cutting surface can be oriented

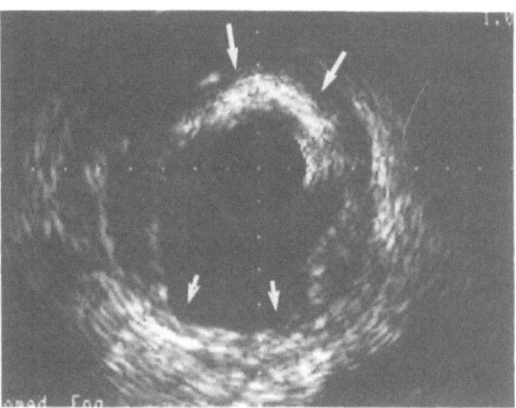

Fig. 2. Ultrasound image from a human iliac artery post atherectomy. The catheter is the dark circle at the center of the grid; calibrations are 1 mm. The atherectomy cut extends into the vessel wall inferiorly (small arrows) but is stopped superiorly by a cap of calcified plaque (large arrows). On the sides of the lumen there is residual soft atheroma 1–2 mm thick.

precisely according to the ultrasound images.

We have found that once the ultrasound images are oriented, interpretation of the images is relatively straightforward, even for operators who are not extensively experienced with ultrasound. The ease of interpretation is no doubt facilitated by the fact that there is only one imaging plane – a cross section, perpendicular to the catheter tip. The hypoechoic appearance of media in most cases (see Fig. 4) is also an extremely useful guide to the location of the true vessel wall. We find that the operators are easily able to assimilate a conceptual three-dimensional representation of plaque morphology by combining information from the ultrasound scans and the tactile and visual feedback of catheter position from the fluoroscope. Subsequent review of the images is problematic in this respect, however, since there is no means at present for indexing catheter position in the recordings of the ultrasound images.

Representative studies

Examples of ultrasound images from two representative cases are shown in Figs. 2–4. In general, our pilot investigations confirm observations from pathologic studies that the amount of atheroma

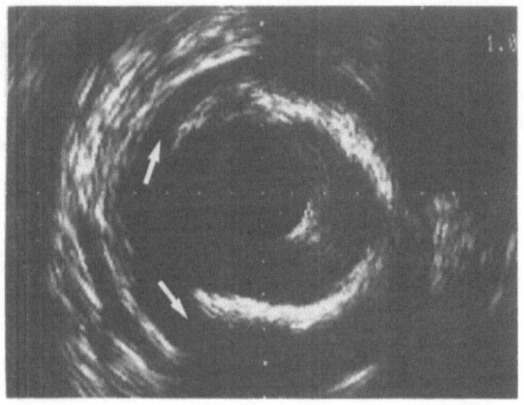

Fig. 3. Dissection in an iliac artery (same patient as above). At this location in the vessel there is a horseshoe-shaped plaque which is attached at its base to the vessel wall to the right. The arms of the plaque have torn loose both superiorly and inferiorly, creating a dissection plane (arrows).

present in the peripheral vessels greatly exceeds what would be predicted based on the angiographic findings. The distribution of the atheroma within the wall is also frequently unpredictable from the angiogram. In Fig. 4B, for example, the deposit of soft atheroma is eccentric, with one wall of the vessel being relatively normal. The angiogram at this level gives no clue either to the presence of atheroma or to the asymmetric deposition in the vessel wall.

The post-atherectomy images demonstrate the same general phenomena: more atheroma is retained following the procedure than would be anticipated on the basis of the angiogram, and the distribution of the residual plaque cannot be determined from the angiographic images. In general, we have found that the post-atherectomy lumen is relatively smooth and that the lumen dimensions correlate with the measurements made by biplane quantitative angiography. The position of the neolumen created by atherectomy, however, may not be centered relative to the vessel wall. The lumen may extend into media on one side of the vessel, but leave a substantial margin of atheroma on the other sides (Fig. 2, 4C).

Imaging has demonstrated a tendency of the Simpson device to preferentially cut soft, as compared to calcified, atheroma (Fig. 2). This property of the catheter was suspected on the basis of clinical performance, and is currently being addressed with advanced designs for cutting. Imaging may be useful in helping to identify those regions of plaque that will require a more aggressive device.

In several cases we were able to identify dissections which were not apparent angiographically. Figure 3 shows one case in which a small dissection developed proximal to the atherectomy site, perhaps due to stretching of the adjacent wall by the action of the balloon on the atherectomy housing. This region was addressed by subsequent atherectomy cuts, and one arm of the plaque was trimmed.

In sections of normal vessel the wall appears remarkably thin compared to regions where atheroma has accumulated (Fig. 4A). All of the atherectomy devices are stated to have selectivity for diseased versus normal vessel wall based on the elasticity of the normal tissue. This selectivity cannot be absolute, however, and it seems fairly clear that imaging orientation may be extremely useful as attempts are made to debulk vessels more aggressively and precisely.

Future technical and clinical directions

The highest priority for current development efforts in ultrasound imaging is further improvement in image quality. The catheters we have tested have sufficiently good image characteristics that discriminating normal from abnormal vessel wall is relatively straightforward for the trained operator. Further improvements in resolution and gray scale, however, should make this process still easier, and allow for more subtle distinctions (such as differentiating thrombus from soft plaque).

The second major technical priority is to make the catheter imaging devices increasingly easy to use. To this end the catheters must have excellent performance characteristics, including flexibility and tracking capability. For work in the coronary arteries it is essential that over-the-guidewire systems be successfully implemented. Perhaps the most significant – and difficult – technical challenge is in attempting to combine imaging and atherectomy in a single catheter. The ability to directly guide the cutting device to regions of atheroma deposi-

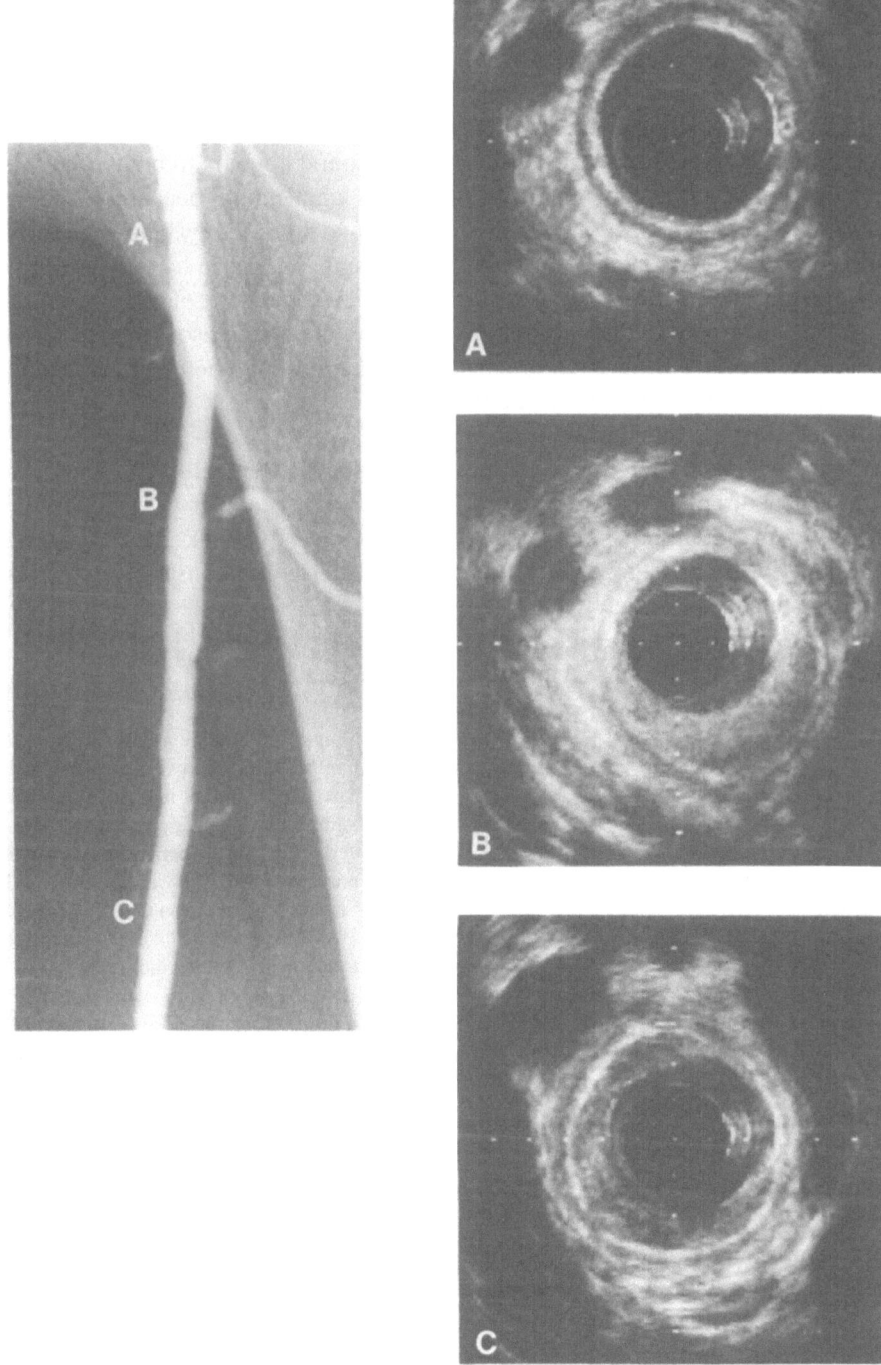

Fig. 4. Angiogram and ultrasound images from a human superficial femoral artery post atherectomy (clinical study). Ultrasound scans are from the positions indicated on the angiogram. *Scan A* shows minimal intimal thickening, with a large, regular lumen. Note the characteristic dark layer corresponding to media. In *Scan B,* there is eccentric plaque deposition most prominent between 2 and 7 o'clock. The medial layer is present but thinned. *Scan C* is from the level of the atherectomy site, which was previously occluded. Despite a relatively good angiographic result, the ultrasound image shows substantial residual atheroma (the neolumen approaches the true vessel wall between 1 and 3 o'clock).

tion would potentially have a major impact in making atherectomy a truly fail-safe and effective microsurgical technique.

A great deal work remains in understanding the clinical implications of the ultrasound images in the context of atherectomy. The basic assumption that extensive debulking of atheroma guided by imaging will provide more favorable long-term results than 'blind' atherectomy needs to be rigorously tested. The rates of acute complications (particularly perforations) with and without imaging guidance need to be established. The imaging technique should provide an answer to the question of whether exposure of media during atherectomy leads to higher restenosis rates. It will also be of considerable interest to determine whether it is possible to remove too much material from the vessel wall from a structural standpoint – that is, whether a thin layer of atheroma should be retained in order to provide support to the vessel wall in regions where the media is extremely thin.

Imaging should also be of considerable use in testing the relative efficacy of the different atherectomy devices. This information may provide a triage strategy for selecting devices. Long regions of concentric atheroma might best be approached with a coaxial device, for example, while eccentric collections would be more effectively removed with a directional device. Possibly the choice of an atherectomy approach in the first place – as opposed to balloon angioplasty, stenting, and so on – can be determined from morphologic features of the vessel wall seen on the ultrasound image. There are preliminary data from the work of Waller and colleagues, for example, suggesting that lesions with a moderate amount of calcification respond more favorably to balloon angioplasty than lesions with either minimal calcium deposits or lesions with large aggregates of calcium [13].

Tissue characterization methods may provide more specific information about the composition of atheroma than is available from imaging alone, and may refine efforts to choose therapeutic methods based on lesion characteristics.

Conclusions

Early experience with the use of intravascular ultrasound imaging as a guide to atherectomy suggests that this new imaging modality may be very useful in allowing maximal debulking of atheroma while decreasing the risk of vessel perforation. Ultrasound appears to be particularly well suited for this application because of the ability to show plaque morphology below the surface of the vessel. Imaging may also be very useful in helping define the relative merit of the different atherectomy devices in comparison to balloon angioplasty and other newer catheter-based technologies.

Acknowledgements

We wish to thank Barbara Herz for her skilled assistance in manuscript preparation.

References

1. Simpson JB, Selmon MR, Robertson GC et al. Transluminal atherectomy for occlusive peripheral vascular disease. Am J Cardiol 1988; 61: 96G–101G.
2. Simpson J, Hinohara T, Selmon M et al. Comparison of early and recent experience in percutaneous coronary atherectomy. J Am Coll Cardiol 1989; 13: 108A (abstract).
3. Selmon M, Robertson G, Hinohara T et al. Factors associated with restenosis following succesful peripheral atherectomy. J Am Coll Cardiol 1989; 13: 13A (abstract).
4. Kensey KR, Nash JE, Abrahams C, Zarins CK. Recanalization of obstructed arteries with a flexible, rotating tip catheter. Radiology 1987; 165: 387–9.
5. Fourrier JL, Auth D, Lablanche JM, Brunetaud JM, Gommeaux A, Bertrand ME. Human percutaneous coronary rotational atherectomy: Preliminary results. Circulation 1988; 78: II–82 (abstract).
6. Stack RS, Perez JA, Newman GE et al. Treatment of peripheral vascular disease with the transluminal extraction catheter: results of a multicenter study. J Am Coll Cardiol 1989; 13: 227A (abstract).
7. Dorros G, Sachdev N, Lewin R, Mathiak L. The acute outcome of atherectomy in peripheral arterial obstructive disease. J Am Coll Cardiol 1989; 13: 108A (abstract).
8. Personal communication, T. Hinohara, M.D.
9. Pinkerton C, Simpson J, Selmon M et al. Percutaneous coronary atherectomy: early experiences of multicenter trial. J Am Coll Cardiol 1989; 13: 108A (abstract).

10. O'Neill WW, Bates ER, Kirsh M et al. Mechanical trans-luminal coronary endarterectomy: Initial clinical experience with the Auth mechanical rotary catheter. J Am Coll Cardiol 1989; 13: 227A (abstract).

11. Hoefling B, Backa D, Bauriedel G, Staeblein A, Jauch KH, Arnim TV. Angioscopic controlled percutaneous atherectomy. Circulation 1987; 76: IV–232 (abstract).

12. Yock PG, Linker D, Saether O et al. Intravascular two-dimensional catheter ultrasound: Initial clinical studies. Circulation 1988; 78: II-20 (abstract).

13. Waller BF, Miller J, Morgan R, Tejada E. Atherosclerotic plaque calcific deposits: An important factor in success or failure of transluminal coronary angioplasty (TCA). Circulation 1988; 78: II–376 (abstract).

International Journal of Cardiac Imaging **4**: 127–133, 1989.
© 1989 *Kluwer Academic Publishers.*

Laser ablation and the need for intra-arterial imaging

C. Borst[1], R. Rienks[2], W.P.T.M. Mali[3], L. van Erven[1]
[1] *Department of Cardiology, Heart-Lung Institute;* [2] *Interuniversity Cardiology Institute of the Netherlands;*
[3] *Department of Radiology, University Hospital Utrecht; Catharijnesingel 101, 3511 GV Utrecht, The Netherlands*

Abstract

In 48 patients with severe claudication due to a total obstruction of the femoropopliteal artery, percutaneous recanalization was attempted with a 2.2 mm diameter rounded sapphire contact probe in conjunction with a continuous wave Nd:YAG laser. In eight patients the contact probe laser catheter took a subintimal course that could not be redressed. Laser recanalization needs high-resolution diagnostic information on the complex anatomy of the obstruction. Intra-arterial ultrasound imaging may provide the necessary information to evaluate, monitor or guide novel angioplasty techniques. The design of an ultrasound catheter which combines high-resolution diagnostic imaging with steerability, flexibility and controlled ablation is now the major engineering challenge in interventional cardiology.

Introduction

Recanalization of arteries by catheter (percutaneous angioplasty) was initiated in 1964 by Dotter and Judkins [1] who used catheters of incremental diameter to widen peripheral artery stenoses. Since the introduction of the balloon catheter in the human coronary arteries by Grüntzig [2] in 1977, balloon angioplasty has become a well established non-surgical treatment of ischemic vascular disease. Balloon dilatation of coronary arteries is being performed in nearly 200,000 patients per year in the US only and it is remarkably effective in reestablishing a hemodynamically adequate lumen [3]. The primary success rate is about 90–95% in experienced centers [3]. However, the procedure has limitations some of which are inherent to its mode of action, overstretching of the wall and fracturing of the plaque [4]. The main limitations are inability to traverse total occlusions, acute thrombotic occlusion (5%) and gradual restenosis in the first six months after the intervention (20–50%) [3].

To address these problems an astounding number of alternative catheter methods have been de-veloped in the past few years [5, 6]. Two approaches are used: stenting the dilated segment [7] or physically removing the obstructing plaque [8–10]. The former approach is guided adequately by fluoroscopy. The latter approach requires more detailed information on the anatomy of the obstructed artery. Plaque removing catheters include mechanical devices which cut [8] or shave [9] and thermal devices which burn [10] their way through the obstruction.

In our hands [11], like in other studies [12, 13], experimental laser angioplasty using bare fibers resulted in perforation of the coronary wall (Fig. 1). Prior to the introduction of the sapphire contact probe in the department [14–17], an attractive method to reduce the risk of perforation was considered to be intra-arterial ultrasound imaging to guide laser ablation using a set of ultrasound crystals positioned in a circle on the rim of the catheter that carried the silica fiber [18, 19]. Bom and co-workers [20, 21] have developed an echo-imaging catheter that employs a single rotating echo element. The need for an imaging catheter is illustrated by the experience with percutaneous laser recanalization of peripheral arteries.

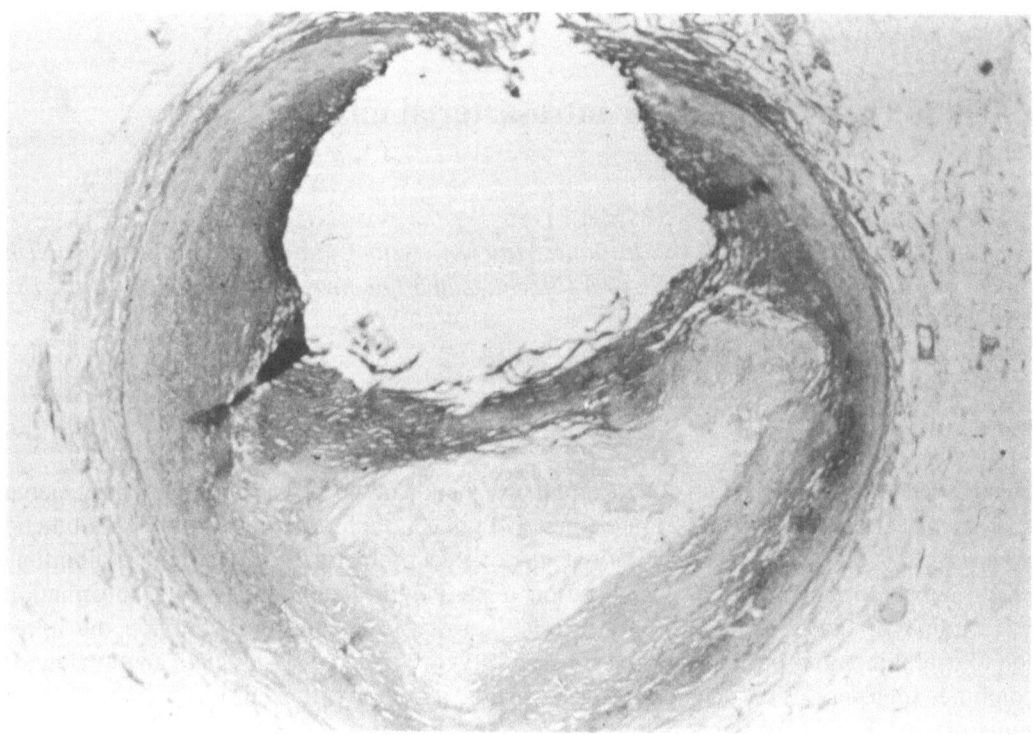

Fig. 1. Result of in vitro attempt at bare fiber (0.6 mm core) recanalization of totally occluded atherosclerotic human coronary artery. The lumen of the laser channel interrupts the external elastic lamina. Note the mixed composition of the fibro-fatty obstruction and the local thinning of the media.

Methods

Forty eight patients with severe claudication due to a total obstruction in the femoropopliteal artery were treated with laser recanalization followed by balloon angioplasty. Details of clinical histories, treatment and early and late results will be reported elsewhere [17]. In brief, a 2.2 mm diameter rounded sapphire contact probe catheter (MRT 1.5, Surgical Laser Technologies, Malvern, PA, USA) (Fig. 2) was used in conjunction with a continuous wave Nd:YAG laser (Medilas-2, MBB, München, FRG, modified [22]; or CL-60, Surgical Laser Technologies, Malvern, PA, USA) as described earlier [15, 23]. The catheter was introduced antegradely in the groin and advanced until resistance required application of 1 s laser pulses. The spot size on front of the sapphire was 1 mm, the power density was 12 W.mm^{-2}.

Results

In the great majority of patients, up to 20 cm occlusions in the femoropopliteal artery were recanalized successfully. In 8 of 48 patients, however, the occlusion could not be traversed. This was not caused by the failure to pass beyond the occlusion. The problem was caused by the fact that the catheter did not reenter the distal lumen after passing the occlusion. During passage through the occlusion the sapphire apparently took a subintimal course or perforated the vessel wall completely. We were unable to differentiate with certainty between these two conditions. Comparison of the left and the right half of figure 3 illustrates that the catheter has taken a subintimal course beyond the distal end of the occlusion. In most of the patients in whom recanalization failed it was possible to advance the catheter subintimally but even with curved catheters we were unable to reenter the lumen (Fig. 3, right).

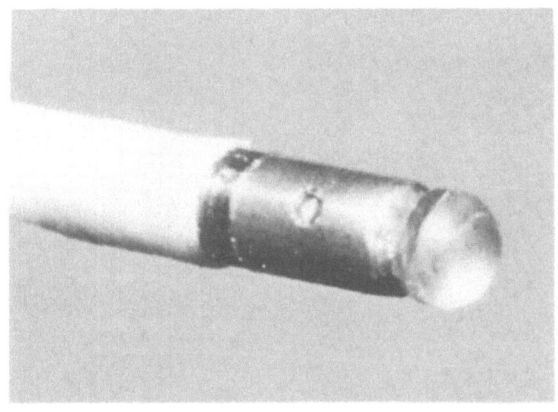

Fig. 2. Laser catheter with 2.2 mm diameter rounded sapphire contact probe (Surgical Laser Technologies).

Discussion

In the femoropopliteal arteries, the low risk of mechanical or thermal perforation (about 10% or less) and the high primary success rate (about 80%) of the metal laser probe [24] and the sapphire contact probe in conjunction with a Nd:YAG laser [17, 25] is to be attributed in part to the atraumatic, blunt shape of these modified fiber tips [5, 15, 23, 26]. The sapphire tip delivers its energy preferentially in the forward direction with limited heating of the lateral side of the sapphire [15, 26]. The 'blind' tracking of the occluded artery on advancing these probes may be attributed to fatty plaque liquefaction, to some preferential thermal ablation of plaque vs normal wall [27] and to the relative resistance to heat of the internal elastic lamina [28]. A mechanical dilatation effect [1] seems to make an essential contribution to the safe and effective recanalization of the femoropopliteal artery because the sapphire tip could traverse, without activating the laser, up to 20 cm long total occlusions in one third of the patients treated in our institute [17].

Unfortunately, the catheter may take a subintimal course and it sometimes fails to reconnect with the distal lumen (Fig. 3). A small diagnostic ultrasound catheter with an imaging plane perpendicular to the vessel axis [20] could show how to reach the distal vessel lumen. However, real-time guiding of laser ablation by catheter ultrasound imaging [18, 19] might prevent taking a subintimal

course from the start. When calcific deposits are present, the current laser catheter will deviate because the laser beam cannot ablate calcifications.

The femoropopliteal artery is serving as the testing ground for novel devices that are to be used ultimately in the coronary arteries. Most devices seem to work quite well in the femoropopliteal artery [5] and perforation is a minor complication. However, the dynamic anatomy of the coronary arteries makes its percutaneous recanalization considerably more difficult and hazardous than the procedure in the upper leg. In particular, the complex anatomy of coronary obstructions forms a basic problem in ablative angioplasty.

The distribution of atherosclerotic plaque is highly variable and its composition is wildly heterogeneous [29–35]. The extent of plaque formation is variable and unpredictable, both in the axial and in the radial direction, although bifurcations and other places where streamline flow is disturbed, or low shear regions are present, are well known predilection places [32]. An excentric stenosis is more common than a concentric stenosis [29, 30] and its lumen may be lined in part with an almost normal wall [29]. Consequently, ablation of the plaque requires careful aiming at a selected part of the cross-section of the artery. In extensively diseased segments of the coronary artery, often little, i.e. less than 100 micron remains of the media (Fig. 1) [29, 33].

A number of diagnostic imaging or sensing modalities have been studied to evaluate their usefulness in guiding plaque ablation: angioscopy, laser fluorescence spectroscopy, electrical tissue impedance and ultrasound imaging.

Angioscopy

Laser ablation guided by angioscopy has been clinically tested by Abela et al. [28] in the femoropopliteal artery. The major limitations to angioscopic guidance are [28, 36]: angioscopy requires displacement of blood by a clear fluid, the information is limited to the visual appearance of the surface and in the coronary arteries proper visualization of the target area is difficult.

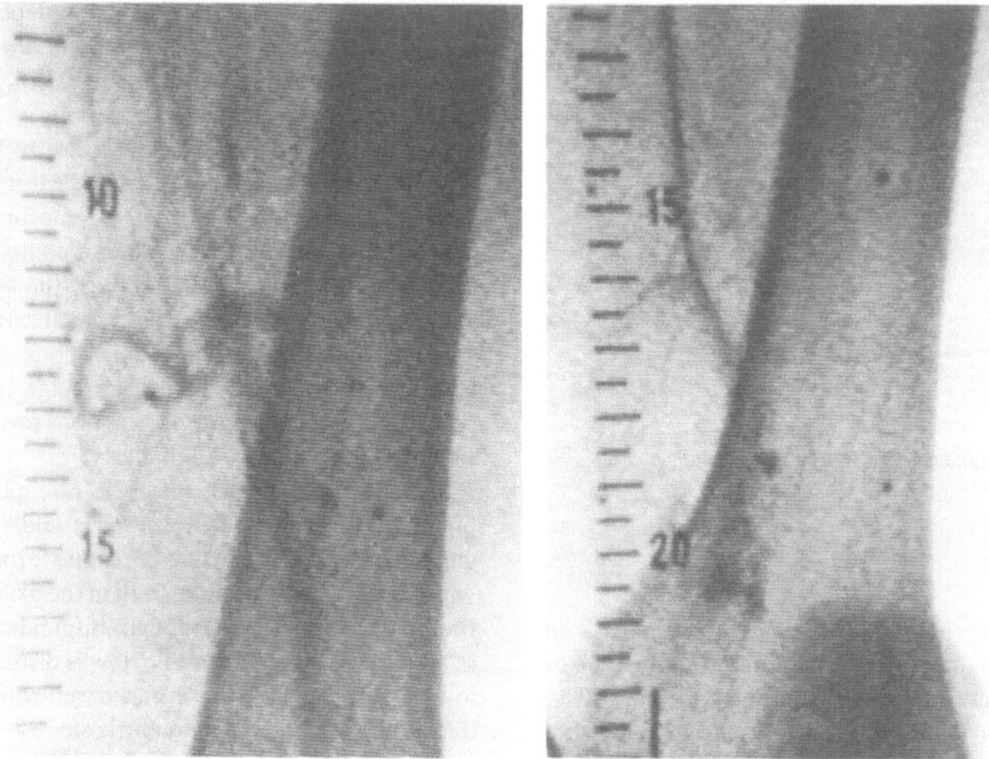

Fig. 3. Left: occlusion in the femoropopliteal artery ends at 11.5 cm. Right: headhunter catheter is advanced to 17.5 cm without entering the open lumen of the distal vessel.

Laser fluorescence spectroscopy

The potential of atheroma identification by laser fluorescence spectroscopy was recognized soon after the initial experiments on laser angioplasty [37–40]. The same silica fiber can be used to transmit the low power excitation laser beam, receive the fluorescent signal and transmit the high power ablative laser beam. Using a HeCd laser (325 nm) for excitation and a pulsed dye laser (480 nm) for ablation, Geschwind et al. [41] achieved promising results in 31 patients with a total occlusion of the superficial femoral artery. However, compared to metal probe [24] or sapphire probe [17, 25] recanalization, the 'smart' approach to laser angioplasty is time consuming. Spectroscopic discrimination of plaque from normal vessel wall may be ambiguous because blood modifies the spectroscopic signals, laser ablation degrades the spectral signature of plaque and plaque composition is heterogenous.

The information is derived from fluorescence of the superficial 50–100 micron layer. Since the media of a heavily diseased coronary artery may be virtually absent [29, 33] (Fig. 1), ablation guided by laser fluorescence spectroscopy may bring the catheter close to the adventitia. Consequently, the catheter may easily perforate during mechanical attempts to refind tissue that is sensed as plaque [41].

The arterial wall elements that discriminate normal wall and plaque by their laser-induced fluorescence signature are elastin and collagen, respectively, according to a preliminary report by Laifer et al. [42]. In arteries the relative collagen/elastin content of normal media and atherosclerotic plaque is 0.5 and 7.3, respectively [42]. However, the fluorescence signal from a thin media [33] is likely to be confounded by the collagen signal from the subjacent adventitia. It is to be noted, however, that no laser induced perforations were reported in the first 31 patients treated with fluorescence guided pulsed laser angioplasty of occluded femoral arteries [41]. In the coronaries, plaque recognition by laser-induced fluorescence spectroscopy is feasible [43], but its value and safety for guided laser ablation remains to be established.

A second possible limitation deserves comment. Successful balloon angioplasty of coronary arteries is followed in 20–50% of cases by angiographic restenosis within the first half year [3, 44, 45]. Its causes are subject to debate [44], but its substrate is now well defined. It often consists of fibrocellular intimal hyperplasia in native arteries [29, 34, 46–50] as well as in saphenous vein bypass grafts [51]. When it contains elastin, laser-induced fluorescence spectroscopy might be incapable of discriminating intimal hyperplasia and normal wall. Restenosed lesions may be even more variable in composition [46–50] and they might generate confusing fluorescence signals.

Electrical tissue impedance

Differentiating atherosclerotic plaque from normal wall on the basis of local differences in electrical tissue impedance [52] is being evaluated as guiding modality for electrical spark erosion [52, 53].

Intra-arterial ultrasound imaging

The development of intra-arterial, real-time, high-resolution, two-dimensional echo-imaging has shown rapid progress in Rotterdam [20, 21] and elsewhere [54–60]. The striking quality of the cross-sectional images allows discrimination of three wall layers which seem to correspond to the intima (echo-dense), the media (echo-lucent) and the adventitia (echo-dense). Atherosclerotic plaque is easily identified. Local wall thickness can be measured acurately as well as the luminal cross-sectional area. Calcific deposits are well delineated but leave echo shadows of doubt about what is behind them. Thus, intra-arterial ultrasound imaging provides unique high-resolution diagnostic information to evaluate or monitor ablation by laser or other modalities.

To advance one more step, to achieve real-time, ultrasound-guided laser ablation, several issues warrant attention. First, laser ablation may generate vapour bubbles which degrade the echo image. Secondly, diagnostic information about the tissue in front of the catheter is badly needed. Thirdly, the current echo catheters are sensitive to deviation from the vessel axis and to movement relative to the wall. Fourth, pulsed laser ablation is usually effected in contact mode. Finally, the incorporation of laser ablation into most of the current rotating single element ultrasound catheters [20, 21, 54–58, 60] may be technically more demanding than incorporating it into a phased-array ultrasound catheter [18, 19, 59].

Conclusions

Intraluminal ultrasound imaging shows promise as guiding modality for emerging catheter recanalization methods, provided no vapour bubbles are generated.

The design of an ultrasound catheter that incorporates imaging and diagnostic features, as well as flexibility, steerability and the capability for controlled ablation, is now the major engineering challenge in interventional cardiology.

Acknowledgements

This work was supported by the Netherlands Heart Foundation (Grants nr. 34.001 and 37.007). We thank professor E.O. Robles de Medina, MD, P.W. Westerhof, MD, S.N. Berengoltz-Zlochin, MD, J.P.J. van Schaik, MD and R.M. Verdaasdonk, MSc for their contribution to the clinical program and Mrs. A.I. Diepeveen for typing the manuscript.

References

1. Dotter CT, Judkins MP. Transluminal treatment of arteriosclerotic obstruction: description of a new technique and a preliminary report of its application. Circulation 1964; 30: 654–70.

2. Grüntzig AR. Transluminal dilatation of coronary artery stenosis (letter). Lancet 1978; i: 263.

3. Bourassa MG (Chairman). Report of the Joint International Society and Federation of Cardiology/World Health Organization Task Force on Coronary Angioplasty. Eur Heart J 1988; 9: 1034–45.

4. Castaneda-Zuniga WR, Formanek A, Tadavarthy M, et al. The mechanism of balloon angioplasty. Radiology 1980; 135: 565–71.

5. Borst C. Percutaneous recanalization of arteries: status and prospects of laser angioplasty with modified fibre tips. Lasers Med Sci 1987; 2: 137–51.

6. Baim DS, guest editor. Interventional Cardiology – Proceedings of a Symposium, June 1987, Sonoma, California. Am J Cardiol 1988; 61: 1G–117G.

7. Sigwart U, Puel J, Mirkovitch V, Joffre F, Kappenberger L. Intravascular stents to prevent occlusion and restenosis after transluminal angioplasty. N Engl J Med 1987; 316: 701–6.

8. Simpson JB, Selmon MR, Robertson GC, Cipriano PR, et al. Transluminal atherectomy for occlusive peripheral vascular disease. Am J Cardiol 1988; 61: 96G–101G.

9. Hansen DD, Auth DC, Hall M, Ritchie JL. Rotational atherectomy in normal canine coronary arteries: preliminary report. J Am Coll Cardiol 1988; 11: 1073–7.

10. Ginsburg R, Wexler L, Mitchell RS, Profitt D. Percutaneous transluminal laser angioplasty for treatment of peripheral vascular disease. Clinical experience with 16 patients. Radiology 1985; 156: 619–24.

11. Rienks R, Straks W, Jambroes G, Hitchcock JF, et al. Possible uses of laser radiation in the treatment of atherosclerotic coronary artery disease. Ned Tijdschr Geneesk 1986; 130: 830–5.

12. Crea F, Fenech A, Smith W, Conti CR, et al. Laser recanalization of acutely thrombosed coronary arteries in live dogs: early results. J Am Coll Cardiol 1985; 6: 1052–6.

13. Isner JM, Donaldson RF, Funai JT, Deckelbaum LI et al. Factors contributing to perforations resulting from laser coronary angioplasty: observations in an intact human postmortem preparation of intraoperative laser coronary angioplasty. Circulation (Suppl II) 1985; II–191–II–9.

14. Borst C, Verdaasdonk RM, Smits PC, Wild D, et al. Laser angioplasty with sapphire contact probe (abstr). Lasers Med Chir (Abstract issue 1st Int Symp Lasers in Cardiovascular Diseases, Baden/Vienna, June 1986), 1986; 6.

15. Verdaasdonk RM, Cross FW, Borst C. Physical properties of sapphire fibre tips for laser angioplasty. Lasers Med Sci 1987; 2: 183–8.

16. Berengoltz S, Westerhof P, Mali W, Verdaasdonk R, et al. Percutaneous transluminal laser recanalization of occluded superficial femoral artery (abstr). Neth J Card 1988; 1: 32.

17. Berengoltz-Zlochin SN, Westerhof PW, Mali WPTM, Verdaasdonk RM, et al. Percutaneous transluminal laser recanalization of occluded femoropopliteal arteries. Ned T Geneesk 1989 (in press).

18. Webster WW Jr. Catheter for removing arteriosclerotic plaque. International Publication Number WO 85/00510 (International filing date patent application: 29 March 1984) PCT/US84/00474.

19. Borst C. Laser Project: Intra-vascular Echo. Project proposal, Utrecht, 11 February 1985.

20. Bom N, Lancee CT, Slager CJ, de Jong N. Ein Weg zur intraluminären Echoarteriographie. Ultraschall 1987; 8: 233–6.

21. Roeland JR, Serruys PW, Bom N, Gussenhoven EJ, et al. Intravascular real-time, high resolution two-dimensional echocardiography (abstr). J Am Coll Cardiol 1989; 13 (Suppl A): 4A.

22. Verdaasdonk RM, Frank F, Borst C. Diaphragm in cavity for low output power application of 100 W Nd:YAG laser. In: G Wollenek, G Laufer and E Wolner (eds), Lasers in Cardiovascular Diseases, Medizinischer Verlag EBM&MZC, München, 1987; pp 37–40.

23. Borst C, Verdaasdonk RM, Boulanger LHMA, Oomen A, et al. Comparison of hot tip and sapphire tip recanalization. In: G Biamino and GJ Müller (eds), Advances in Laser Medicin I, Ecomed, Landsberg/Lech, 1988; 70–80.

24. Sanborn TA, Cumberland DC, Greenfield AJ, Welsh CL, Guben JK. Percutaneous laser thermal angioplasty: initial results and 1-year follow up in 129 femoropopliteal lesions. Radiology 1988; 168: 121–5.

25. Lammer J, Karnel F. Percutaneous transluminal laser angioplasty with contact probes. Radiology 1988; 168: 733–7.

26. Verdaasdonk RM, Rienks R, van Erven L, Borst C. Sapphire and metal tip recanalization: implications for safety. In: GJ Müller, ed. Advances in Laser Medicin III. (In press).

27. Welch AJ, Valvano JW, Pearce JA, Hayes LJ, Motamedi M. Effect of laser radiation on tissue during laser angioplasty. Lasers Surg Med 1985; 5: 251–64.

28. Abela GS, Seeger JM, Barbieri E, Franzini D, et al. Laser angioplasty with angioscopic guidance in humans. J Am Coll Cardiol 1986; 8: 184–92.

29. Becker AE, Anderson RH. Cardiac Pathology. Churchill Livingstone, Edinburgh, 1983; Chapter 3, pp 3.1–3.11.

30. Hangartner JRW, Charleston AJ, Davies MJ, Thomas AC. Morphological characteristics of clinically significant coronary artery stenoses in stable angina. Br Heart J 1986; 56: 501–508.

31. Small DM. Progression and regression of atherosclerotic lesions. Insights from lipid physical biochemistry. Arteriosclerosis 1988; 8: 103–9.

32. Glagov S, Zarins C, Giddens DP, Ku DN. Hemodynamics and atherosclerosis. Arch Path Lab Med 1988; 112: 1018–31.

33. Almagor Y, Leon MB, Bartorelli AL, Lenhard SD, et al. Media thinning of severely diseased coronary arteries: guidelines for new interventional procedures (abstr). J Am Coll Cardiol 1989; 13 (Suppl A): 194A.

34. Von Pölnitz A, Backa D, Nehrlich G, Höfling B. Histological evaluation of 'Vessel-Biopsies' obtained with the Simpson atherectomy catheter (abstr). J Am Coll Cardiol 1989; 13 (Suppl A): 149A.

35. Ross R. The pathogenesis of atherosclerosis – an update. N Engl J Med 1986; 314: 488–500.

36. Grundfest WS, Litvack F, Hickey A, Doyle L, et al. The current status of angioscopy and laser angioplasty. J Vasc Surg 1987; 5: 667–73.

37. Kittrell C, Willett RL, de los Santos-Pacheo C, Rattliff NB, et al. Diagnosis of fibrous arterial atherosclerosis using fluorescence. Appl Opt 1985; 24: 2280–1.

38. Leon MB, Lu DY, Prevosti LG, Macy WW Jr, et al. Human arterial surface fluorescence: atherosclerotic plaque identification and effects of laser atheroma ablation. J Am Coll Cardiol 1988; 12: 94–102.

39. Laufer G, Wollenek G, Hohla K, Horvat R, et al. Excimer laser-induced simultaneous ablation and spectral identification of normal and atherosclerotic arterial tissue layers. Circulation 1988; 78: 1031–9.

40. Clarke RH, Isner JM, Gauthier T, Nakagawa K, et al. Spectroscopic characterization of cardiovascular tissue. Lasers Surg Med 1988; 8: 45–59.

41. Geschwind HJ, Dubois-Randé JL, Poirot G, Boussignac G. Guided percutaneous pulsed laser angioplasty: results and follow up (abstr). J Am Coll Cardiol 1989; 13 (Suppl A): 13A.

42. Laifer LI, O'Brien KM, Stetz ML, Gindi GR, Deckelbaum LI. Etiology of the fluorescence difference between normal and atherosclerotic arteries (abstr). Circulation 1988; 78 (Suppl II): II–448.

43. Bartorelli AL, Almagor Y, Prevosti LG, Swain JA, et al. In vivo coronary plaque recognition by laser-induced fluorescence spectroscopy (abstr). Circulation 1988; 78 (Suppl II): II–294.

44. McBride W, Lange RA, Hillis LD. Restenosis after successful coronary angioplasty. Pathofysiology and prevention. N Eng J Med 1988; 318: 1734–7.

45. Nobuyoshi M, Kimura T, Nosaka H, Mioka S, et al. Restenosis after successful percutaneous transluminal coronary angioplasty: serial angiographic follow-up of 229 patients. J Am Coll Cardiol 1988; 12: 616–23.

46. Essed CE, Van den Brand M, Becker AE. Transluminal coronary angioplasty and early restenosis: Fibrocellular occlusion after wall laceration. Br Heart J 1983; 49: 393–6.

47. Giraldo AA, Esposo OM, Meis JM. Intimal hyperplasia as a cause of restenosis after percutaneous transluminal coronary angioplasty. Arch Path Lab Med 1985; 109: 173–5.

48. Austin GE, Ratliff NB, Hollman J, Tabey S, Phillips DF. Intimal proliferation of smooth muscle cells as an explanation for recurrent coronary artery stenosis after percutaneous transluminal coronary angioplasty. J Am Coll Cardiol 1985; 6: 369–75.

49. Ueda M, Becker AE, Fujimoto T. Pathological changes induced by repeated percutaneous transluminal coronary angioplasty. Br Heart J 1987; 58: 635–43.

50. Morimoto S, Sekiguchi M, Endo M, Horie T, et al. Mechanism of luminal enlargement in PTCA and restenosis: a histopathological study of necropsied coronary arteries collected from various centers in Japan. Jpn Circ J 1987; 51: 1101–15.

51. Saber RS, Edwards WD, Holmes DR Jr, Vlietstra RE, Reeder GS. Balloon angioplasty of aortocoronary saphenous vein bypass grafts: a histopathologic study of six grafts from five patients, with emphasis on restenosis and embolic complications. J Am Coll Cardiol 1988; 12: 1501–9.

52. Bom N, Slager CJ, Phaff A. Sensing methods for selective recanalization by spark erosion. Proc IEEE/9th Ann Conf Eng Med Biol Soc, 1987; pp 205–6.

53. Slager CJ, Essed CE, Schuurbiers JCH, Bom N, et al. Vaporization of atherosclerotic plaque by spark erosion. J Am Coll Cardiol 1985; 5: 1382–6.

54. Yock PG, Johnson EL, Linker DT. Intravascular ultrasound: development and clinical potential. Am J Cardiac Imag 1988; 2: 185–93.

55. Bartorelli AL, Potkin BN, Almagor Y, Gessert JC, et al. Intravascular ultrasound imaging of atherosclerotic coronary arteries: an in vitro validation study (abstr). J Am Coll Cardiol 1989; 13 (Suppl A): 4A.

56. Pandian N, Kreis A, O'Donnell T, Sacharoff A, et al. Intraluminal two-dimensional ultrasound angioscopic quantitation of arterial stenosis: comparison with external high-frequency ultrasound imaging and anatomy (abstr). J Am Coll Cardiol 1989; 13 (Suppl A): 5A.

57. Linker DT, Johansen E, Sloerdal S, Yock PG, et al. In vivo measurement of segmental arterial wall stiffness in pigs using a real-time ultrasonic sector imaging catheter (abstr). J Am Coll Cardiol 1989; 13 (Suppl A): 218A.

58. Tobis JM, Mallery JA, Mahon D, Griffith J, et al. Intravascular ultrasound visualization of atheroma plaque removal by atherectomy (abstr). J Am Coll Cardiol 1989; 13 (Suppl A): 222A.

59. Graham SP, Brands D, Savakus A, Hodgson JMcB, et al. Utility of an intravascular ultrasound imaging device for arterial wall definition and atherectomy guidance (abstr). J Am Coll Cardiol 1989; 13 (Suppl A): 222A.

60. McKay C, Waller B, Gessert J, Collins S, et al. Quantitative analysis of coronary artery morphology using intracoronary high frequency ultrasound: validation by histology and quantitative coronary arteriography (abstr). J Am Coll Cardiol 1989; 13 (Suppl A): 228A.

International Journal of Cardiac Imaging **4**: 135–143, 1989.

3-D visualization of arterial structures using ultrasound and Voxel modelling

Richard I. Kitney, Lincoln Moura & Keith Straughan
Bio-Medical Systems Group, Department of Electrical Engineering, Imperial College, London SW7 2BT, UK

Summary

In this paper, a new type of vascular imaging system is presented which is designed for use in conjunction with percutaneous transluminal treatment techniques (balloon and laser angioplasty, atherectomy etc). Three dimensional computer models of arterial sections are reconstructed in full voxel space from data acquired using a purpose-built, catheter-mounted ultrasound probe. The system is standalone, using commercially available computer hardware and specially written software. The software is equally compatible with source data from other modalities (e.g. CT and MR), and the system can therefore be incorporated into a PACS environment.

Introduction

Over the last few years it has become apparent that the amount of information which is contained in various types of lesions is simply too large and too detailed to be conveyed in written or tabular form. While it is true that some imaging modalities have been available for some considerable time, for example conventional X-rays on film, it has only been with the advent of the digital computer and mass storage media that image manipulation has become possible.

The study of arterial disease over recent years has been specifically based on the use of ultrasound. The assumption on which ultrasonic scanners are based is that the plaque can be seen using B-mode imaging, and/or detected from velocity disturbances arising from its formation. However, arterial structures and plaque are, almost by definition, three dimensional. Hence 3-D imaging of such structures is seen as a worthwhile goal in its own right. More specifically, improved imaging techniques may reduce the unpredictable risk that remains during balloon and laser angioplasty, related to damage to the intimal surface of the vessel.

Currently, it is impossible to obtain adequate information in realtime about the effect of these procedures. Conventional contrast radiographic techniques provide intermittent images with poor visualization of the intimal surface. Fibre-optic angioscopy improves resolution, but requires complete obstruction to blood flow.

3-D space and object description

Over the last few years there has been increasing interest in the use of computer graphics to represent and manipulate 3-D objects. The main strategies employed have been to represent the object in the form of either a wire or solid model. From a technical standpoint the first option is far easier to implement, but for many applications it is relatively unrealistic. Hence, an increasing amount of work has been undertaken on the development of computer-based solid models of 3-D objects. Such modelling strategies are based on three approaches: Constructive Solid Geometry, Boundary Representation or B-rep, and Voxel Space Modelling.

Constructive solid geometry – CGS modelling

CGS modelling is based on the fact that man-made objects can be built using simple geometric shapes. In CGS these basic shapes are called primitives and objects are represented by sets of operators, for example union and intersection, applied to primitives positioned by means of translation and rotation. Figure 1 illustrates a chess pawn generated using this approach. The number of parameters required to define each primitive is dependent upon its geometry. However, each primative usually requires three co-ordinates for its centre plus three angles of rotation. A sphere requires an additional value, its radius, while a cylinder requires two parameters, for radius and length.

Since CGS objects are defined as conglomerates of primitives, any operation performed on an object must be performed on each of its constituent parts and the relative positions of each of the components maintained. This operation can be assisted by determining the intersection between a plane and the 3-D model. In CGS modelling this intersection is calculated by finding the intersection between every primitive and the given plane.

CGS models must be computed each time they are used. Computing intersections and unions between primitives is very time consuming, hence the processing time grows not only as a function of the number of primitives, but, even more significantly, as a function of the number of interactions between primitives. Figure 2 shows a CGS model of a carotid artery simulation using approximately 160 primitives organised in the form of rings.

CGS modelling forms the basis of a large number of CAD/CAM packages where man-made objects are to be modelled. However, CGS is not a good approach to the 3-D modelling of anatomical or many biological structures because of the large number of geometric primitives which are required.

Boundary representation (B-rep)

The B-rep approach to 3-D modelling is a very natural one as it is closely related to the methods

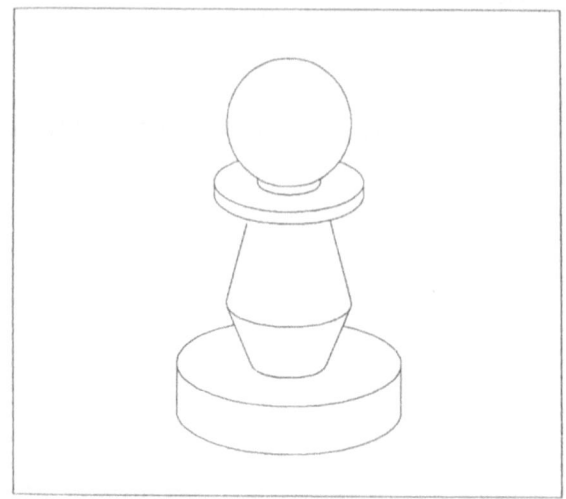

Fig. 1. A constructive solid geometry chess pawn.

used in 2-D drawing. In the 2-D case a curve is represented by a sequence of x, y points connected in the simplest form by a straight line or lines. Boundary Representation is a direct extension of this concept to the 3-D case. In the 3-D situation volume is defined by surfaces which delimit it. The surfaces are described by sets of points (x, y, z) which are connected, again in the simplest form, by straight lines. However, whereas in the 2-D case the sequence of points gives the order of connection, here such a simple connection cannot be implemented since any point on the boundary surface is connected to more than one other point. Hence the connection order must be explicitly given by using either explicit polygons, explicit edges or by keeping a list of points and their connections. Usually the region within the polygons on the model surface is assumed to be planar ie a facet, hence the method may be referred to as B-rep, or faceted.

Data input to Boundary Representation systems is usually performed by either defining a series of contours in different planes and then allowing the system to connect them, or by defining primitives in a similar manner to that used in Constructive Solid Geometry. In the latter case models are not stored as CGS models, but as facets and vertices computed from the primitives as they are defined. Boundary representation is very suitable when the structures to be modelled are smooth ie when not

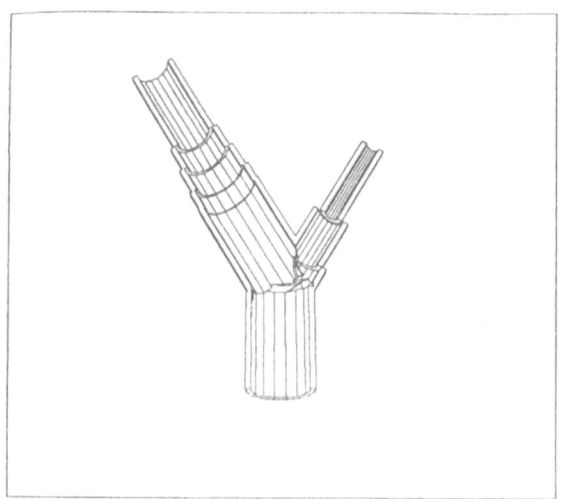

Fig. 2. A CGS Carotid Artery Simulation with nearly 160 blocks in the complete segment.

too many facets are required to represent the volume adequately.

Performing any operation on a B-rep model means processing all the facets individually. For boundary representation models, finding the intersection between a given plane and the 3-D model implies finding the intersection between the plane of each facet and the intersecting plane. If the intersection occurs within the facet, then the intersection line must be computed, otherwise the facet is not intersected by the plane. For models with many facets this operation is very time consuming.

The strength of the boundary representation method lies in the fact that it uses computer memory as required, hence simple models are accurately represented by small amounts of memory. This subsequently leads to fast processing. This is one of the basic reasons why boundary representation is so popular with 3-D modelling packages designed for microcomputers. Since B-rep models are represented by their boundary surfaces, which in turn are made of facets, it is necessary that each facet be oriented in order to convey the information both 'inside' and 'outside' the volume. This is usually done by keeping track of the direction of the vector normal to each facet, assumed to point outwards from the model [1].

Boundary representation models are defined by lists of vertices, their connections and normal vector directions. These lists must be kept in very strict order. If for any reason a single value in any of these lists is suppressed, or even modified, the resulting model will bear little or no resemblance to the original model. Using B-rep it is possible to define models which cannot be defined in the real world such as the famous Escher objects [2]. Most of the CAD/CAM systems which are currently available make use of boundary representation in order to define the solid model. Historically, B-rep models were the first to be implemented on computers, and consequently most of the theory and the computer techniques developed for the handling and viewing of 3-D models were initially developed using B-rep objects. An example of a B-rep rendering from our work on carotid bifurcations is illustrated in Fig. 3.

Voxel modelling

In the Voxel Space approach the 3-D space is divided into Nv cubes called voxels arranged side by side as illustrated in Fig. 4. A voxel v can be defined by the co-ordinates of its centre (x, y, z), where x, y and z are assumed to be integers in the interval [1, N_v]. Hence, voxel space VS is defined by:

$$VS = \{V/1 \leq x \leq N_v \wedge 1 \leq y \leq N_v \wedge \leq z \leq N_v\} \quad (1)$$

where the symbol { denotes The Set Of, / denotes so that, and $\wedge$ denotes the Boolean operator And.

An interesting feature of Voxel Space representation is that it always represents volumes, as opposed to surfaces. As a consequence Voxel-Space models are always physically consistent.

A number V(v) associated with each voxel is called the 'voxel value' or 'voxel content' and can be used to determine whether a voxel is part of an object. In its simplest form a voxel v may be said to pertain to an object O if V(v) is non-zero ie

$$0 = \{v/V(v) \neq 0 \wedge \in VS\}$$

where the symbol $\in$ stands for In.

138

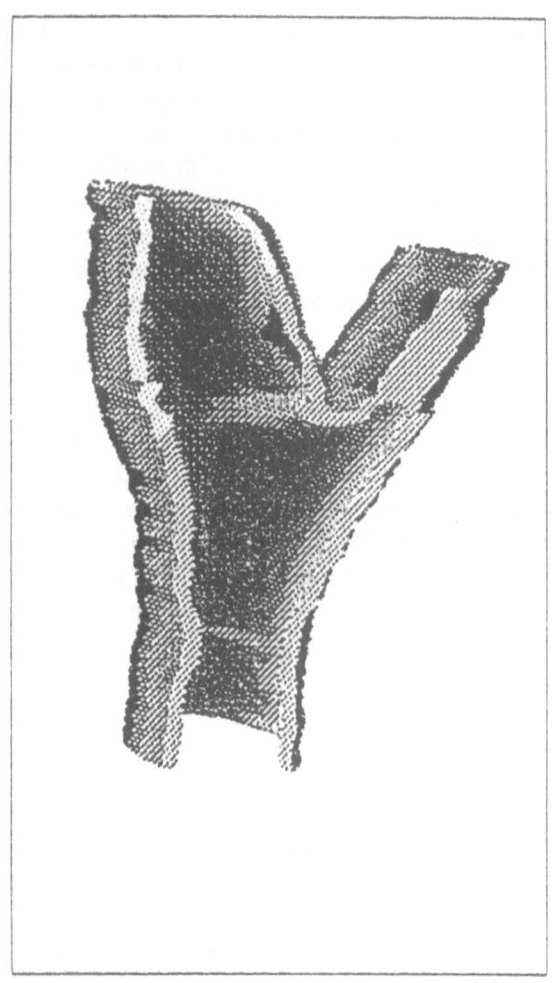

Fig. 3. A B-rep carotid bifurcation simulation.

The voxel, or volume element, can be considered as an extension to 3-D space of the digital image element or pixel (picture element). Indeed, the Voxel Space can be represented by a 3-D array in the same manner as the digital image is represented by a 2-D array. Any plane of the voxel space can be seen as a digital image. In particular, a plane defined by z = k – called a voxel plane – can be associated with a digital image D as follows.

$$D(x, y) = V(x, y, x) \qquad (2)$$
$$1 \leq x \leq N_v, \Lambda 1 \leq y \leq N_v, \Lambda z = k$$

where $D(x, y)$ is the pixel value at the pixel (x, y) on the image D and $V(x, y, z)$ is the voxel value at the

Voxel Space co-ordinates (x, y, z). This concept is illustrated in Fig. 4. The analogy between voxels and pixels will not be discussed in any more detail here, it is sufficient under the present circumstances to view Voxel Space as an environment which resembles cubic images.

Voxel space representations tend to be extremely computer intensive because the number of voxels required to define complex, lifelike objects is large. In fact the number of voxels in Voxel Space – the voxel space resolution – determines the model complexity. Even though objects can be encoded in order to reduce the amount of memory required to store them, the processing time is ultimately dependent on the number of voxels in the Voxel Space.

Although the use of Voxel Space representation is relatively new when compared with boundary representation (the concept of Voxel Space was first applied in the mid 70's [3] and its use for medical purposes began seriously in 1979 (Herman and Liu), a considerable amount of effort has now been applied to Voxel space representation, giving good results.

Voxel modelling of arterial structures

Let us assume that a 2-D image of an arterial cross-section is represented by M × M picture elements or pixels. This concept can be extended to the imaging of three dimensional objects. The depth, or z dimension, of the object can be constructed from a series of 2-D pixel planes by laying them one behind the other.

The 2-D picture elements (pixels) now become cubes. These cubes, which form the 3-D image, are called volume-elements or voxels. Hence a 3-D object can be modelled in M × M × N voxel space.

Our current software, which produces full voxel space images, allows display and manipulation in both 2-D and 3-D, with the ability to easily transfer from one to the other [4, 5]. The design of the system also allows a wide range of operations to be performed on 3-D solid models. These include: rotation in all three dimensions; cross-sectional displays at any depth; shaded images using depth

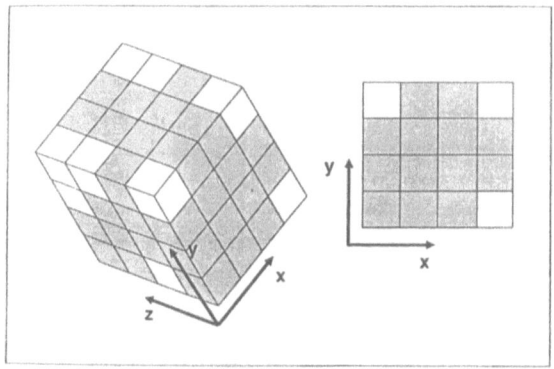

Fig. 4. The voxel plane and digital images. Any voxel plane can be seen as a digital image. In particular, voxel planes parallel to the X–Y plane can represent series of square images taken at different depths.

code; plane cuts so that any section of the model can be removed; and X-ray projection – where a 3-D structure can be made semi-transparent.

Using voxel models, a series of 2-D arterial slices can be used to produce a 3-D image. We have developed an alternative approach which is to acquire parallel 2-D slices from the artery under examination using a catheter-mounted ultrasonic probe. The 2-D morphological information obtained in this way is converted into a 3-D solid model of the section of artery under investigation. The time taken to acquire the data is small in comparison to the cardiac cycle, hence the slices can be aligned without significant movement error.

Contour definition

If a single arterial slice is imaged in terms of N sets of polar co-ordinates, then each contour can be described by:

$$R(i), \theta(i) \quad \text{for} \quad i = 1\text{-----}n$$

where $R(i)$ is the radius from the centre of the image plane and $\theta(i)$, the corresponding angular direction.

On the basis of this information, for any given slice, a contour can be drawn which corresponds to a change in acoustic impedance. Multiple contours

are similarly calculated. The information for a single slice is now contained in 2-D pixel space. This process is repeated N times to generate the slices which form the 3-D arterial volume. If the pixel space comprises $M \times M$ pixels, then the volume consists of $M \times M \times N$ voxels. This information is then used to construct a solid model of the arterial section.

3-D Interpolation

One interpolation strategy is to assume that the radii vary linearly between the original slices. Consider the case where, for example, there are three slices separated in the digital scene in such a way that they correspond to the planes 10, 30 and 50. (The overall voxel space again being $M \times M \times N$.) It is necessary to calculate the contours for planes 11 to 29, and 31 to 49. In order to do this it is assumed that any given radius will vary linearly between any two original consecutive slices ie

$$R(m, j) = \quad (3)$$
$$\frac{(m - m_0)}{(m_1 - m_0) \times (R(m_1, j) - R(m_0, j))} +$$
$$R(m_0, j) \text{ for } m = m_0 + 1, m_1 - 1$$

where m is the mth slice to be calculated, m_0 is the position of the nearest 'below' original slice, and m_1 the nearest 'above' original slice. If equation (3) is now applied to the linear interpolation problem previously defined, then we have:

$$R(m, j) = \quad (4)$$
$$\frac{(m - 30)}{(50 - 30) \times (r(50, j) - R(30, j))} + R(30, j)$$

Figure 5 illustrates an example of the Voxel Space software being used to reconstruct a model from a series of pathological slices. Referring to the Figure, the bottom left section shows one of the original photographs which was frame-grabbed. The illustration above (top left), shows the same section following initial enhancement, for example back-

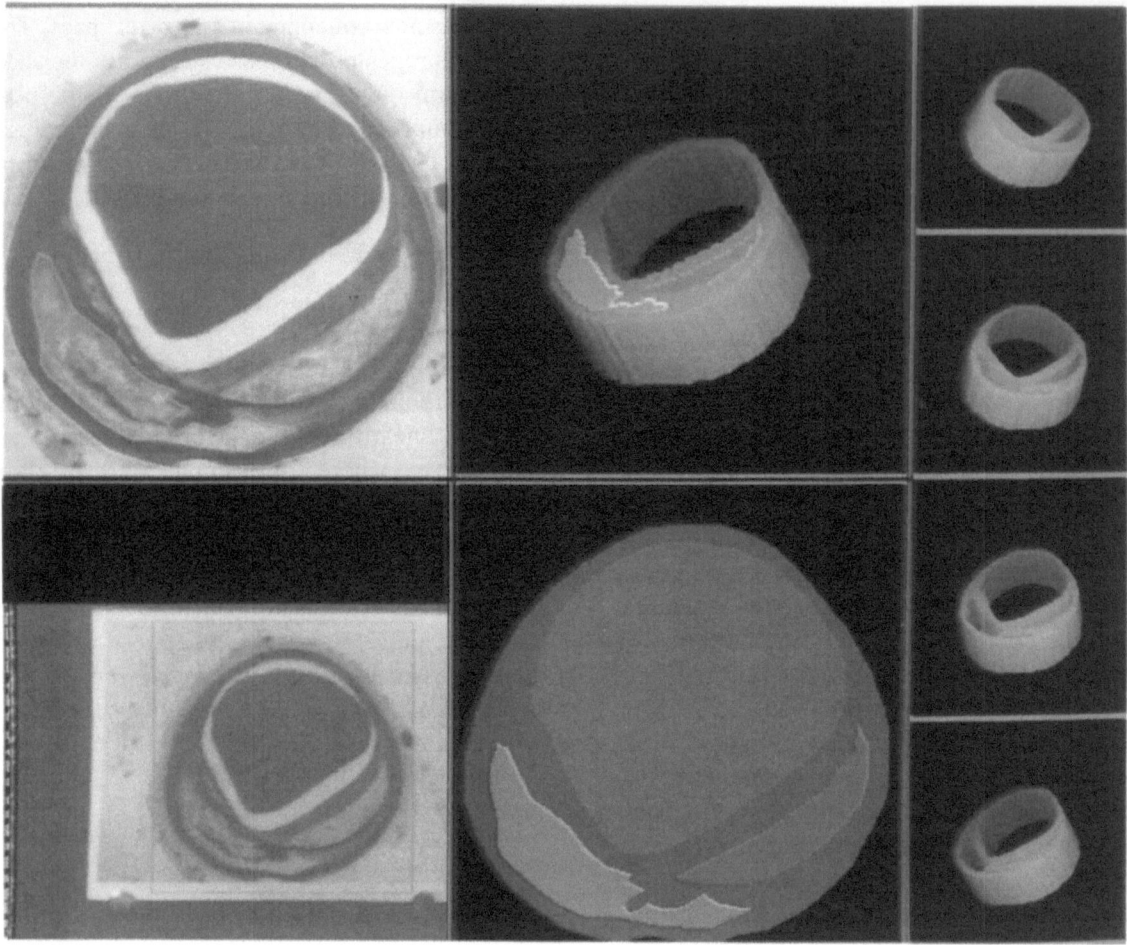

Fig. 5. Construction of voxel model of an arterial section from a sequence of pathological slices.

ground equalisation. Careful inspection of the figure reveals that the outer arterial wall is now identified by a closed contour (orange), as are two sections of tissue within the lumin (blue and green contours). This was done for the purpose of tissue characterisation and can be more clearly seen in the colour version of the cross-section (bottom right). The top right illustration shows the 3-D voxel model which in this case has been reconstructed from a sequence of 10 pathological slices. The column of four illustrations on the right of the figure show the model in different orientations with the identified tissue sections removed. These sections (blue and green) are now voxel models in their own right and can be examined independently. The example shows the significant potential of the system in the field of tissue characterisation. Such characterisation can also be carried out using the ultrasound probe (described later). It is important to note that a key factor in the use of ultrasound in the study of arterial disease is its ability to visualise the internal structure of the arterial wall. This is course is impossible with straight visual inspection techniques.

3-D visualisation of arterial structures using ultrasound

System description

We have developed a standalone ultrasonic system for the 3-D visualisation of arterial sections. The system comprises a catheter mounted phased array which is connected to a specially designed ultrasonic transceiver capable of operating between 6 and 20 MHz. The ultrasonic transceiver is interfaced with a Microvax II computer (a 32 bit machine with a 40 MHz clock). The associated graphics terminal is a Sigmex 6244 with a resolution of 1448 × 1024 (vertical) pixels with a palette of 256 colours.

Results

The results which will be discussed illustrate 3-D reconstructions of data obtained from three sources. Firstly, 'phantom' data measured directly from models of diseased arteries were used to test the software. 2-D slices of the model are reliably recreated by the computer (Fig. 6). Using this series of 2-D slices, the software reconstructs a 3-D model in full voxel space (Fig. 7).

Secondly, data were collected from postmortem tissue using the ultrasonic probe. These were used to reconstruct 3-D computer models of the original specimens. Fig. 8 illustrates a section of normal carotid artery reconstructed in 3-D using ultrasonic data obtained from the catheter-mounted probe. In figure 8B a section of the artery has been removed by the software, revealing the intimal surface of the vessel.

Figure 9 demonstrates additional software capabilities of the system. Here a section of normal femoral artery has been reconstructed from ultrasonic data acquired from inside the artery using our specially designed catheter. Fig. 9A shows a low resolution model which is used for very rapid rotation; Fig. 9B is the full resolution version of Fig. 9A; Fig. 9C is 9B in transparent mode, showing contours of a potential oblique cut; and Fig. 9D is the full resolution version of 9C.

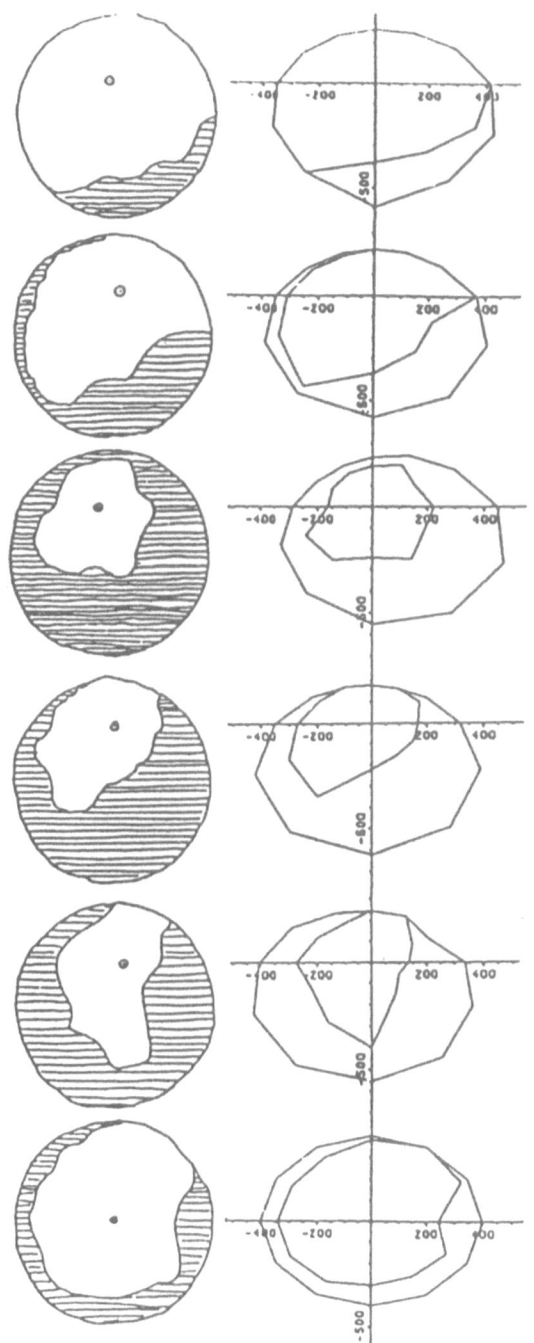

Fig. 6. A series of 2-D slices from a hardware phantom of a diseased artery (left column) is reliably reconstructed by the software (right column).

142

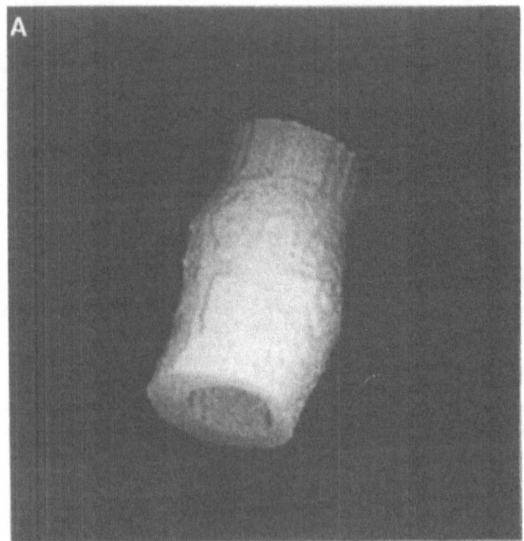 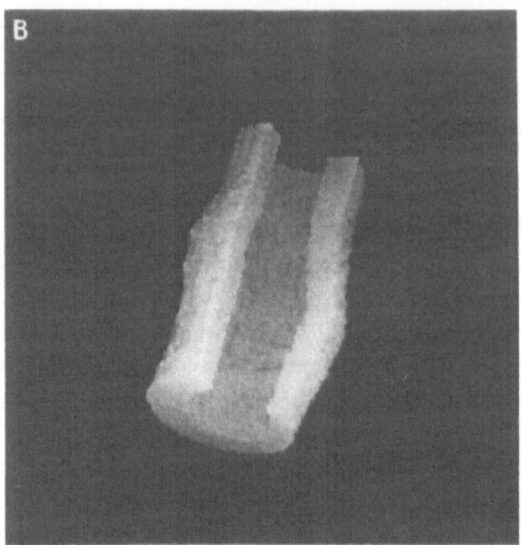

Fig. 7. A 3-D reconstruction of a normal carotid artery from ultrasonic data. Figure 7B shows a section of the arterial wall removed by the software.

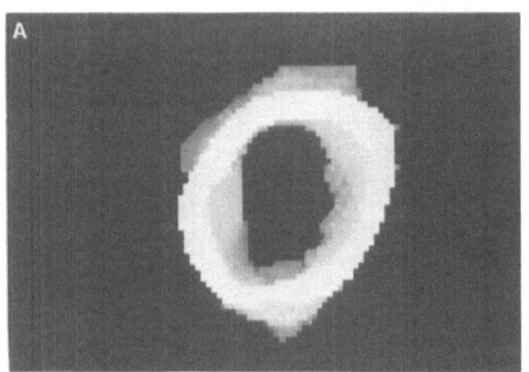 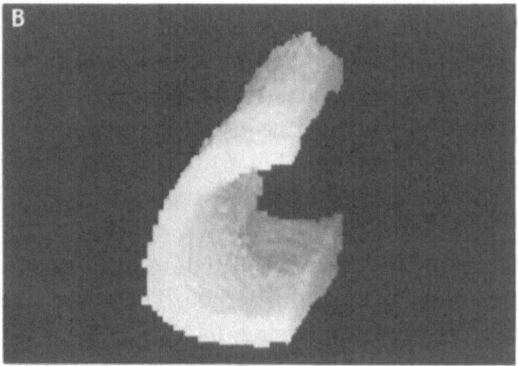

Fig. 8. A 3-D reconstruction of atheromatous aorta from ultrasonic data. Figure 8A is an end-on view, while Fig. 8B shows the arterial section in a different orientation with a section of the wall removed by the software to allow easier examination of the plaque.

Discussion

In this paper we have reviewed the application of 3-D computer based modelling techniques to the visualisation of arterial structures. Of the various modelling methods which are available, constructive solid geometry, boundary representation and voxel space, the latter is seen as being the most appropriate for the modelling of anatomical structures. The principal reasons for this are: (a) voxel modelling can easily accommodate highly irregular structures; (b) the technique is able to describe the internal features of the lumin in great detail (as opposed to only the surface features, as would be the case for B-rep); (c) voxel modelling is truly digital and hence allows the rapid construction of 2-D images from the 3-D visualisation in any orientation.

The incorporation of the 3-D modelling software which we have developed, into a special purpose ultrasonic imaging system, has resulted in the ability to obtain high resolution images. The current system works virtually in realtime and we expect to have a truly realtime system fully operational within 3 to 4 months.

The research presented in this paper therefore

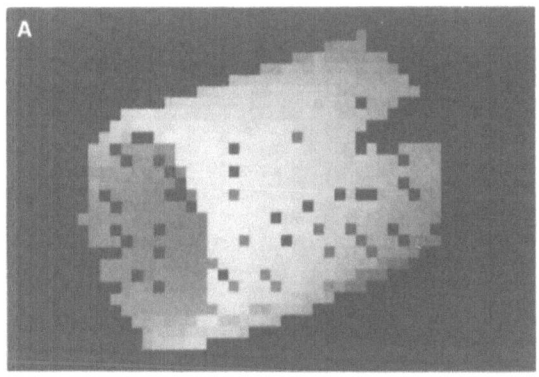
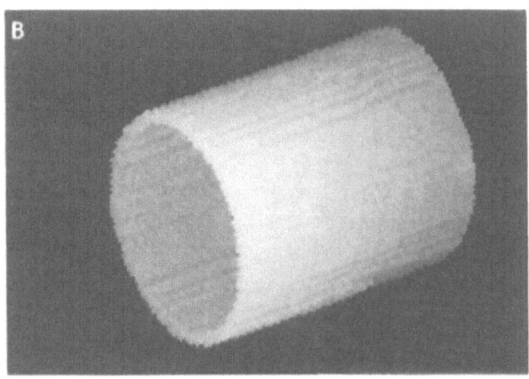
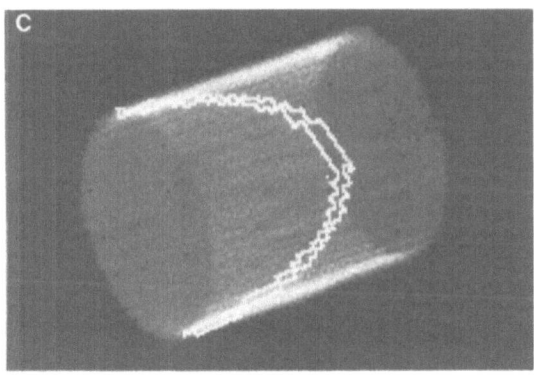
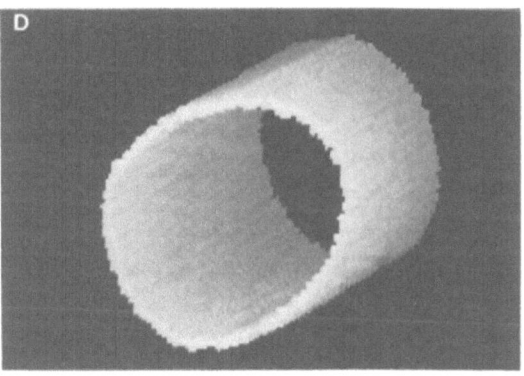

Fig. 9. A 3-D reconstruction of a section of normal femoral artery from ultrasound data, recorded in-vivo. Figure 9A, a low resolution model which is used for rapid rotation; Fig. 9B, the full resolution version of Fig. 9A. Fig. 9C, Fig. 9B in transparent mode showing the contours of a potential oblique cut, and Fig. 9D the full resolution version of 9C.

represents a new approach to arterial imaging based upon ultrasound measurements which should be capable of being employed in a wide range of applications.

Acknowledgements

We warmly acknowledge the support of our clinical collaborators: Drs Rothman, Burrell and McDonald of the Cardiac Department, The London Hospital, who have undertaken the clinical aspects of the project.

References

1. Foley JD, van Dam A. Fundamentals of Computer Graphics. Pub. Addison Wesley, 1984.

2. Pipes A. Solid modellers: This year's style. CAD/CAM International, 1985; 9: 20–23.

3. Robb RA et al. 3-D Visualisation of the Intact Thorax and Contents: A Technique for Cross-sectional Reconstruction from X-ray views. Computers and Biomedical Research, 1974; 7: 395–419.

4. Kitney RI, Moura L, Straughan K. Three dimensional modelling of arterial structures using ultrasound. Proc. IEEE. Ninth Annual Conf. of the Engineering in Medicine and Biology Soc. Vol. 1, 400–401, 1987.

5. Kitney RI, Moura L, Straughan K, Burrell CJ, Rothman M, McDonald AH. Ultrasonic Imaging of Arterial Structures using 3-D Solid Modelling. Proc. IEEE Conf. on Computers in Cardiology. Bethesda, Sept 1988. In Press.

6. Farrell EJ. Visual interpretation of complex data. IBM Systems Journal 1987; 26: 174–200.

7. Herman GT, Jayaram KU. Display of 3-D digital images: Computational foundations and medical applications. IEEE Trans C G and A 1983; pp 39–45.

8. Herman GT. Computerised reconstruction and 3-D imaging in medicine. Ann Rev of Comput Science. 1986; pp 153–79.

International Journal of Cardiac Imaging **4**: 145–151, 1989.
© 1989 *Kluwer Academic Publishers.*

Optimized ultrasound imaging catheters for use in the vascular system

R.J. Crowley[1], P.L. von Behren[2], L.A. Couvillon Jr.[1], D.E. Mai[2] & J.E. Abele[1]
[1] Boston Scientific Corporation, Watertown MA, USA; [2] Diasonics Inc., Milpitas, CA, USA

Abstract

Clinical experience with 6 and 9 Fr ultrasound imaging catheters (UICs) reveals that several transducer and catheter tip varieties are needed for optimum imaging of diseased intravascular sites. Our UIC design has combined established catheter design and very high frequency ultrasound imaging technology to create a versatile, user configured system for intravascular ultrasound imaging. Optimum use requires proper strategic selection of transducer and catheter sizes, frequencies of operation, and interventional accessories.

Introduction

New techniques for angioplasty, increasingly prominent in scientific conferences, are currently the subject of much enthusiasm and investment. There has been an accompanying strong interest in imaging modalities and guidance systems which might provide better evaluation of lesion morphology and character than traditional angiography.

Very few of the 'new' angioplasty techniques, or the guidance systems, are genuinely new. There are many references to thermal angioplasty, curretage (atherectomy), stents, electrical ablation, and other currently fashionable topics, in literature more than twenty years old, and patents from the 19th century [1]. Intravascular ultrasound is no exception; Bom has written an excellent historical summary describing work in this area [2]. The tendency of medical innovations to have a very long gestation time was studied in the 1970s by Rushmer [3]. These innovations have a tendency to be periodically rediscovered.

Our work suggests that optimized intravascular ultrasound products must apply the lessons learned over many years about catheter design, ultrasonic imaging, and the needs of the interventionalist.

Motivation

Our own interests in intravascular ultrasound have accompanied our work in balloon angioplasty from its beginning in the early 1970s. Over this period the use of balloons expanded from early pioneers and 'hobbyists' to the clinical mainstream. The barriers to the expansion of angioplasty and related less-invasive techniques have been systematically beaten down over the years, through a collaboration among device innovators and visionary clinicians. To be sure, many of these barriers have been medico-political as well as technological. Technical advances have not guaranteed clinical utility.

A key technical barrier to wider use and improved clinical efficacy of angioplasty, and the fundamental motivation for intravascular ultrasound, is the relatively poor information about vascular disease provided by conventional angiography. Angiographic views are two-dimensional shadowgram projections of contrast-opacified vessels. These two-dimensional images often provide a deficient or misleading representation of the actual three-dimensional vasculature. Lesion morphology and percentage of stenosis are not well quantified. Detailed visualization of anatomy and loose material or flaps is difficult because overlying tissue reduces contrast. The known harmful effects of ionizing radiation, and concerns about osmotic effects of radiographic dyes, restrict the imaging time available. Nevertheless, angiography is currently the diagnostic 'gold standard' for the interventionalist.

Direct optical vision of lesions has been a long-standing dream. It was attempted in the 19th century using various glass tubes [4]. In the 1950s, rigid endoscopes using relay lenses began to appear, and were successful in certain applications where their size and stiffness did not outweigh their benefits. The development of coherent bundles of flexible optical glass fibers in the 1960s and '70s led to the growth of medical endoscopy as a key medical specialty, especially in gastroenterology and pulmonary medicine. Our own work in fiber optic applications resulted in a variety of inexpensive catheter endoscopes known by the name Visicath™* [5].

Optical endoscopes have continued to improve in flexibility and resolution, and to decrease in size, during the 1980s. However, in spite of research enthusiasm, their application in vascular imaging has been limited and problematic. Blood obscures the optical image, and an image from within the lumen of the endothelial surface, although useful, does not provide information about the internal structure and composition of the vessel wall.

External ultrasound can provide detailed, real time pictures of vascular anatomy, including plaque character and location. Doppler ultrasound studies provide information on blood flow. However, external ultrasound is limited by frequency dependent attenuation which restricts its highest useful frequencies to the 10 MHz range and a maximum depth of about 4 cm. The lateral resolution is consequently limited, especially in deeper structures. Another major shortcoming of external ultrasound is that of acoustic access; it is often difficult or impossible to reach a target vessel with ultrasound energy because of an inadequate acoustic path in the overlying tissue. Lack of acoustic access severely limits cardiac studies. Another constraint is vessel tortuosity which makes scanning extended vascular segments difficult because only a small part of the vessel may lie within the thin tomo-

graphic slice of the ultrasound scan. Finally, vessel motion due to cardiac pulsation can move the subject in and out of the scan plane.

Table 1 gives an overview of the advantages and disadvantages of angiography, optical endoscopy, and external and intraluminal ultrasound.

Design evolution

As part of an experimental assessment of excimer laser angioplasty, we concluded that intraluminal ultrasound was more likely to provide suitable anti-perforation guidance than alternatives like emission spectroscopy. To establish feasibility, a 1 mm diameter, 20 MHz air-backed hand-rotated transducer was constructed*, and used with rudimentary imaging electronics to produce images of wire phantoms and tissue samples. These images were crude, but provoked a next step, the objective of which was grey-scale images from a catheter with practical flexibility. We obtained improved 1 mm transducers, mounted them on various shafts, and began a series of in vitro and animal experiments.

Around the time of these initial experiments, the combined excimer laser-ultrasound system was abandoned. Attention was directed to an intra-vascular ultrasound imaging system for diagnosis and intervention with the following overall performance specifications:
- The catheter construction should be modular. Optimum economics are provided by a multi-use transducer within a single-use sheath having a sonolucent 'window' region.
- Numerous catheter designs and accessories must be provided, based on the variety of standard diagnostic catheter shapes and functions which have evolved in interventional medicine, and will continue to evolve.
- The catheter should have acceptable flexibility, torque properties, and feel, and be constructed from approved catheter materials. Generally, it should have performance characteristics already familiar to interventionalists.
- A family of system sizes must be provided: a 6 Fr

* Boston Scientific Corp., Watertown, MA.

* Craig J. Hartey, Houston, TX: personal communication.

initial system for peripheral vessels around 1 cm in diameter; smaller (4 Fr) and/or larger (9 Fr) systems later for coronary vessels or deeper penetration.

- An initial imaging frequency of 20 MHz was selected; the system should be upgradeable to higher (30 + MHz) and lower frequencies later for higher resolution at short range, or longer range.
- Well-established ultrasound electronic technology should be used, to take advantage of existing hardware and software functions applicable to intraluminal imaging, and the existence of a field service infrastructure.

An initial analog display system was constructed for catheter development [6]. Following a period of animal experiments and two clinical trials [7], Boston Scientific Corporation and Diasonics, Inc. formed a cooperative program in which BSC is responsible for the catheters and Diasonics in the electronics. This project has resulted in the BSC Sonicath™ ultrasound imaging catheter, which operates with the Diasonics IVUS™ ultrasound console. This equipment allowed routine, reliable images of diseased arteries to be obtained at several clinical sites (Fig. 1).

Design alternatives

Several types of Sonicath™ UIC designs have been evaluated and are in various stages of commercialization. An even greater variety of optimized sizes, transducers and scan schemes will be available as imaging of more specific lumenal conditions progresses. This leaves the user with choices involving tradeoffs. Understanding the characteristics and limitations of these various catheter configurations will allow the interventionalist a higher probability of successful intravascular ultrasound imaging.

The Sonicath™ has various tip configurations to match its catheter function. It is available with distal floppy tips of various sizes, preformed curves, and in piggyback wire-guided versions. These configurations (Fig. 2) are similar to those of commonly used vascular catheters; the tip configuration affects the utility, but not the imaging properties. All of the tip configurations use the same catheter body and sonolucent window.

Catheter size, however, has a strong influence on imaging performance. There are now three basic size categories of Sonicath™ UICs, all which have performance advantages under certain circumstances. The first is a class of 6 to 7 Fr, 110 cm long

Table 1. Comparison of vascular imaging modalities

Modality	What you see	Advantages	Disadvantages	
Angiography	Two-dimensional shadowgram of opacified vessel – side view	Excellent 'road map' of vessel contour	Shows contour only; Medium resolution; Uses harmful radiation	Fluid pressure hides flaps; Requires potentially harmful contrast agents; Views limited to injection time
Angioscopy	Three-dimensional, axial color view	Good resolution; Excellent view of surface; Color helps definition	Requires injection of clear fluid; Surface images only	Views limited to injection time
External ultrasound	Real time tomographic slice	Non-invasive; Larger organs seen well	Requires acoustic access	Frequency dependent resolution
Catheter ultrasound	Two-dimensional radial cross section ('slice')	Good resolution of small structures; Sees through vessel wall; No fluid injection required – longer real time views possible	Slice views only; Difficult to aim forward	Invasive

148

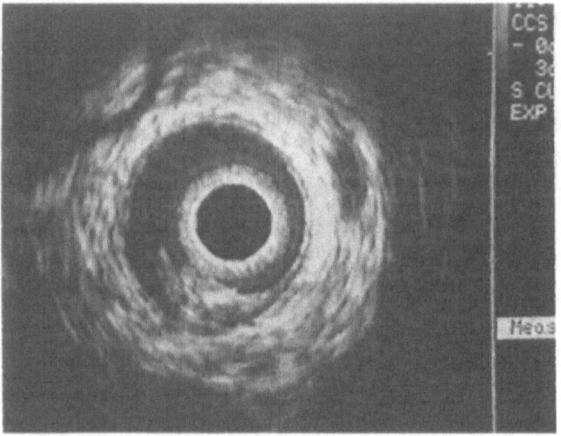

Fig. 1. 6 Fr UIC image of atherosclerotic human iliac artery.

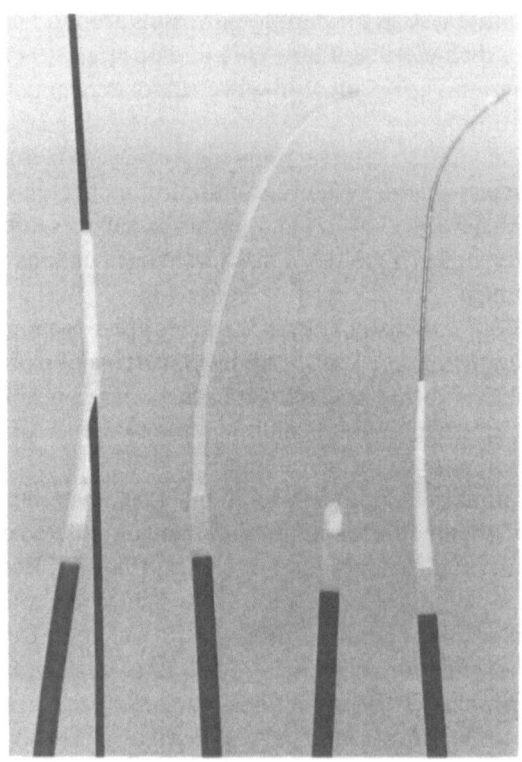

Fig. 2. Selection of UIC tip styles. L–R, 6 Fr. 0.035″ over-the-wire, 6 Fr. 0.035″ covered floppy tip, 6 Fr. round tip, 6 Fr. 0.018″ platinum floppy tip. All versions can be interchangeably used with a single 20 MHz transducer.

catheters that are designed for vessels in the extremities such as the popliteal, femoral and iliac arteries. This size UIC can be placed via introducer sheaths commonly used for catheter access to these sites, or over an 0.035″ guidewire in suitably equipped versions. When tipped with an 0.018″ or 0.035″ distal floppy guidewire, the torque properties of the braided catheter body can be used effectively to manipulate and guide the UIC while lessening the probability of intimal damage.

The second category of UICs includes a larger diameter (9 Fr) version with greater imaging range, for use in the aorta, larger iliac arteries and for intracardiac imaging of valves. The larger transducer aperture allows the use of a lower operating frequency for range extension, or an improvement in resolution at an unchanged frequency. Figures 3 and 4 are a general comparison of arterial images obtained from both 6 and 9 Fr, 20 MHz UICs. Though lateral resolution of both images is good in the near field, at deeper penetration the 9 Fr is clearly superior; a smaller beam spread of small details at a distance of 5 mm and greater is fairly obvious. Axial resolution is virtually the same.

A flexible eyelet at the end of some 9 Fr UIC versions allows the device to be placed and guided over a 0.035″ guidewire to the region of interest. An interesting and possibly important variation in UIC placement involves the use of sonically transparent introducer sheaths that can be positioned

over a guidewire. The guidewire can then be withdrawn and the UIC inserted and advanced and withdrawn through the region of interest, such as aortic and mitral valves. Aside from the repeatability that this method affords, there may be significant safety benefits.

Coronary UICs comprise the third major category. The need for much smaller diameters to negotiate the more tortuous coronary arteries offers significant mechanical and acoustic design challenges. At 3 Fr (1 mm) the maximum practical transducer element aperture is in the range of 0.6 mm. The ratio of catheter wall thickness to element diameter suffers an undesirable decrease. Because of the relatively small aperture, lateral resolution suffers if the transducer center frequency remains at 20 MHz. However, adequate acoustic penetration at 30 MHz has been demonstrated in smaller vessels. Resolution can then be main-

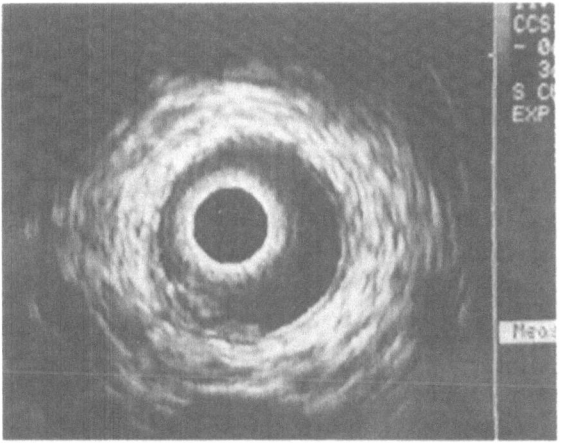

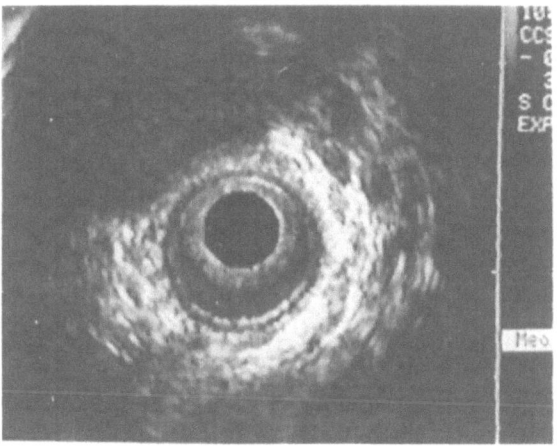

Fig. 3. 6 Fr UIC image of iliac artery. At far field distance, tissue features are seen as curvilinear areas since beam spread increases with distance.

Fig. 4. 9 Fr. UIC image of femoral artery. At far field distance beam spread is less than in 6 Fr. image, resulting in better lateral resolution.

tained, and image quality similar to that of 20 MHz, 6 Fr UICs can be realized.

As catheter size increases, further improvements in image quality can be gained. Catheter wall thickness may not need to increase much from 6 to 9 Fr, but transducer aperture increases significantly. Lateral resolution beyond the near field transition point improves and beam spread decreases markedly, but this is not the only benefit. Much greater effective penetration can be achieved because the radiated power and sensitivity is greater in a larger aperture transducer. We have measured an almost twofold power and sensitivity increase when the transducer aperture is increased from 1 to 1.75 mm in diameter. It follows that the user should select the largest aperture size if best image quality is the primary goal. When practical considerations necessitate the selection of catheters bearing transducers of smaller aperture, careful settings of the imaging electronics can enhance interpretation.

There are several reasons why larger apertures are desirable in some applications (see Figs. 5 a–c). There are also some drawbacks. For a given transmit frequency, a larger aperture emits more sound energy into the tissue resulting in greater penetration. Anatomy further from the transducer, such as adjacent veins, can be visualized. The larger aperture lengthens the near field zone where the lateral resolution is best. However, the lateral

resolution in the near field worsens, since it is proportional to aperture size. The larger transducer aperture allows the use of a lower operating frequency which improves tissue penetration and maintains a longer near field depth. Figure 6 schematically depicts frequency dependent attenuation with depth. Lower frequencies travel a greater distance in tissue than higher ones. When better penetration is desired, lower frequencies and/or more power from larger apertures must be used.

Transducer technology

There are many transducer technologies available for constructing catheter based ultrasound imagers. Possible configurations include mechanically scanned and electronically scanned transducers. Materials such as PZT (lead zirconate-titanate) or PVDF (polyvinylidine fluoride) could be used. Various transducer geometries – flat, curved, circular, annular etc., could be constructed. We chose a mechanically rotated single PZT crystal for several reasons. First, the simplicity of the transducer and signal processing electronics over that of array based systems allows for quicker development cycles for new applications, reduces the cost of the system, and improves reliability. Second, mechanically scanned transducers provide better image

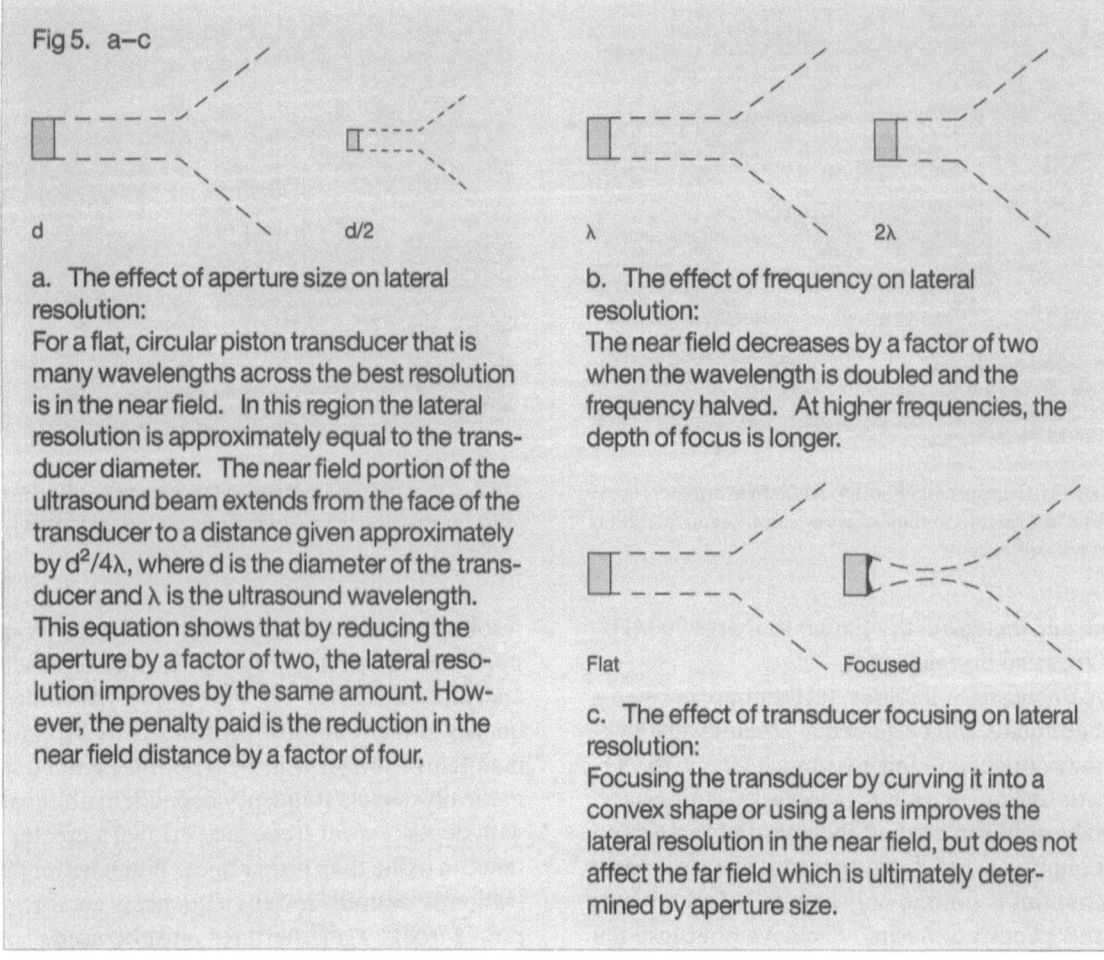

Fig 5. a–c

d   d/2

a. The effect of aperture size on lateral resolution:
For a flat, circular piston transducer that is many wavelengths across the best resolution is in the near field. In this region the lateral resolution is approximately equal to the transducer diameter. The near field portion of the ultrasound beam extends from the face of the transducer to a distance given approximately by $d^2/4\lambda$, where d is the diameter of the transducer and λ is the ultrasound wavelength. This equation shows that by reducing the aperture by a factor of two, the lateral resolution improves by the same amount. However, the penalty paid is the reduction in the near field distance by a factor of four.

λ 2λ

b. The effect of frequency on lateral resolution:
The near field decreases by a factor of two when the wavelength is doubled and the frequency halved. At higher frequencies, the depth of focus is longer.

Flat   Focused

c. The effect of transducer focusing on lateral resolution:
Focusing the transducer by curving it into a convex shape or using a lens improves the lateral resolution in the near field, but does not affect the far field which is ultimately determined by aperture size.

quality than electronic arrays. This is because a mechanically scanned transducer always points a full aperture into the tissue. This allows maximum acoustic power to be transmitted into the tissue, resulting in better penetration and lateral resolution. A curved array geometry results in reduced aperture because only a few elements face the transmit/receive direction. The use of rotating drive cable to very accurately provide a mechanical scan has been shown to be entirely practical, and our experience has shown it to be economical as well.

Future directions

Interventional ultrasound is a new imaging modal-ity still in clinical trials. It is likely to evolve in a fashion similar to external ultrasound. Continually improving image quality will provide ever better diagnostic capabilities. Catheter designs, initially generic and 'all purpose', will continue to become more applications specific and expand into new configurations. All of the scanning modes used by external ultrasound are potentially available to interventional ultrasound. M-mode may be useful for assessment of motions of valves, cardiac chambers and vessel walls. C-scan imaging, using data from forward looking transducers, could provide images of tissue planes perpendicular to the catheter axis. Doppler tipped catheters are currently used to measure blood velocity; the combination of this technology with imaging capability is under development. Color doppler imaging, a hybrid of imag-

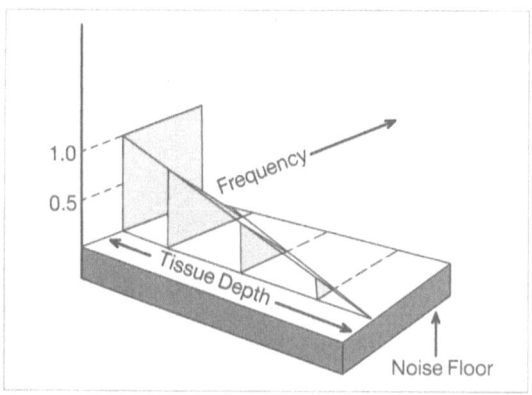

Fig. 6. Schematic depiction of frequency dependent attenuation with depth. Higher frequency sound waves are more quickly absorbed in tissue, and their received echo amplitude decreases more quickly as well. At some limiting depth, information from all frequencies is lost and only noise remains.

ing and Doppler modes, may have applications in evaluating blood flow near vascular lesions.

New display techniques may be developed to better communicate the anatomical and functional information to the clinician. Three-dimensional reconstruction of the vasculature from a sequence of interventional ultrasound images has been demonstrated by Kitney et al. [8]. Multimodality displays will show angiographic, ultrasound and perhaps angioscopic views simultaneously using split video screen techniques.

References

1. Hamilton J.R. Thermal Dilator. United States Patent 1898; No. 612, 724: October 18.
2. Bom N, ten Hoff H, Lancee CT, Gussenhoven WJ, Serruys PW, Salger CJ & Roelandt J. Early and present examples of intraluminal ultrasonic echography. 1989; Proc SPIE 1068.
3. Rushmer RJ, Alternative Futures for Biomedical Research: The ALZA Distinguished Lecture. Presented at Annual Meeting of the Bio-Medical Engineering society, Dallas, TX, April 9, 1979. Annals of Biomedical Engineering 1979; 7: 1–44.
4. Cortis B.S, Harris D.M. & Principe J. From Angiography to Angioscopy: Information Discussion, Texas Heart Journal September 1986; 13: 281–289.
5. Bloch E.C. & Filston F.C. A Thin Fiberoptic Bronchoscope as an Aid to Occlusion of the Fistula in Infants with Tracheoesophageal Fistula. Anesth Analg 1988: 67: 791–3.
6. Ellis R.A., Crowley R.J. & Eyllon M.M. Ultrasonic Imaging Catheter 1988; Proc SPIE 904: 127–30.
7. Crowley R.J. Ultrasound Catheter Imaging. a Functional Overview 1989; Proc SPIE: 1068
8. Kitney R.I., Straughan K. & Moura L. Catheter-mounted Ultrasound Probe for 3-D arterial Reconstruction 1989; Proc SPIE: 1068.

International Journal of Cardiac Imaging **4**: 153–157, 1989.
© 1989 *Kluwer Academic Publishers.*

Intraluminal ultrasound guidance of transverse laser coronary atherectomy

H.T. Aretz,[1] M.A. Martinelli,[2] & E.G. LeDet[2]
[1] *Lahey Clinic Medical Center, 41 Mall Road, Burlington, MA 01805, USA;* [2] *Intra-Sonix, Inc., 42 Third Avenue, Burlington, MA 01803, USA*

Abstract

Catheter systems for laser atherectomy in peripheral and coronary arteries are subject to many design constraints. Ideal mechanical, laser and imaging requirements for these systems are proposed, and compared to the design features of a laser atherectomy system currently under development by Intra-Sonix. This system uses high resolution ultrasound for real-time guidance and control and is potentially capable of characterizing lesions and imaging critical structures in the coronary arteries, to guide physicians in the application of laser therapy. Precise catheter location and rotational direction can be provided continuously as the therapeutic intervention proceeds. Examples are given of the imaging modes and ultrasound images of an artery produced by the Intra-Sonix system.

Introduction

Intravascular ultrasound and laser atherectomy devices have reached the clinical stage as separate entities. Several laser devices have progressed from peripheral to coronary artery applications and are presently in clinical trials. Due to their size (usually greater than 5 F) and stiffness, intraluminal ultrasonic devices are still applied mostly in peripheral vessels. Clinical trials with imaging before and after either balloon angioplasty or mechanical atherectomy have been carried out in the peripheral vascular system, but currently there is no single catheter combining imaging and treatment modalities applicable to either the coronary or peripheral arteries.

In this paper we discuss the rather formidable requirements for an ideal coronary laser atherectomy system in general and the proposed solution to these requirements by the Intra-Sonix laser atherectomy system in particular.

The ideal coronary laser atherectomy system

A coronary laser atherectomy device should combine laser delivery and imaging in a single catheter. It should be small, flexible but torqueable, deliverable over a standard guidewire, and disposable. Imaging should be spatially coincident with the therapy, real-time, and allow characterization of lesions. Ideally the lesions should be debulked and the remaining surface should lead to decreased chronic restenosis without creating significant emboli, vascular spasms or acute thrombosis. Additionally, in order for such a system to be of clinical use, it has to be easy to use and cost-effective.

Catheter mechanics

Minimally, the catheter should be capable of accessing coronary artery lesions now addressable by balloon angioplasty. Because of the difficulty in reaching such treatment sites, the catheter must have a lumen for a guidewire. Even with the use of a guidewire, the catheter and its associated cabling must be highly flexible and probably less than 3 F to reach these therapy sites. The tortuous path through which the device must be steered requires that the catheter be torqueable to provide control and the proper 'feel' to the interventionalist.

Ideally, the catheter should be disposable to eliminate the potential for viral cross-contamination and the sterilization, storage and maintenance requirements that would be associated with a re-usable device. This implies that it be manufactured at a reasonable cost.

Laser

There are several considerations governing the choice of laser delivery and the laser itself. One fundamental question is whether the laser light should be delivered radially, directed at the wall and lesion, or forward, coaxial with the lumen of the artery. If the laser is fired radially, the system cannot be used in total occlusions since the lesion has to be first traversed by a guidewire. Firing radially, however, will allow for a total debulking of the lesion, if adequate imaging is available. We emphasize that these considerations address laser atherectomy, not the use of lasers for opening a passage through total occlusions for introduction of balloon catheters or other therapeutic devices.

For a system that combines ultrasound with the laser, the most likely choice is a pulsed laser which leads to predictable and reproducible ablation of atheromatous tissue, including calcified plaques. The wavelength should be such that it can be delivered through readily available optical fibers. Thermal damage should be minimized and debris should be such that it is inconsequential to the distal circulation. Finally, the surface left behind should lead to less acute and chronic complications than balloon angioplasty, in addition to reducing the all important restenosis rate. A laser that encompasses all of these features has yet to be identified with certainty.

Imaging

The ideal imaging requirements for laser atherec-

tomy are also quite stringent. First, the imaging system should provide a field-of-view that is coincident with the laser radiation, so that the physician has a clear visual representation of the area in which the therapy is being applied. Also, it is highly desirable that the system be capable of real-time imaging so that the effectiveness of the therapy can be monitored while it is in progress.

Of course, the imaging system must provide sufficient image quality that the need and degree of therapy at a candidate site can be determined. This includes both dimensional accuracy and tissue characterization capability for evaluating lesions and making appropriate therapeutic specifications. In addition, image resolution should be good enough to clearly identify critical areas that must be avoided during therapy.

It is important to recognize that therapeutic applications require different image quality considerations than those for diagnostic use. Ponderous image interpretation is inconsistent with the risk and time demands of the therapeutic setting; the image quality must allow for rapid, reliable judgements by the clinician. Therefore, image quality in this sense may involve less (or more localized) information content than that which is common in diagnostic systems, provided that unambiguous decisions can be made quickly.

Acute and chronic arterial effects

Any laser angioplasty or atherectomy system will have to deal with the acute and chronic effects of the therapy. Acutely, there may be spasms, which in laser systems, particularly thermal systems, are associated with the amount of heat applied. There may be acute thrombosis, which is usually related to local dissections or highly thrombogenic surfaces leading to an acute closure of the artery. A much less predictable and troublesome effect is the chronic recurrence of the plaque, in an apparently accelerated fashion, after a period of three to six months. Presently, in one third of all patients who have undergone balloon angioplasty, significant stenoses will recur with significant lesions in that time frame. If laser atherectomy in any form is to be effective, this percentage has to be significantly reduced to justify the probable increased cost of the procedure. It is not clear what the ideal final arterial surface after the procedure should be to avoid chronic arterial effects. It is our belief based on theoretical considerations, in the absence of human data, that laser atherectomy has the ability to significantly reduce the restenosis rate, but this may best be achieved in conjunction with pharmacologic agents.

System description

Application

The Intra-Sonix system is being developed to treat cases of severe (but not total) stenosis in the coronary arteries by laser atherectomy. It uses ultrasound as the imaging modality to guide the physician at the treatment site and monitor the progress of plaque removal during the therapy. The ultrasound has sufficient resolution to characterize the structure of the artery wall and associated pathology.

Design

A diagram of the principal system components is shown in Fig. 1. The ultrasound imaging device and transverse laser delivery means are mounted in a disposable catheter. The precise locations of the ultrasound and laser radiation with respect to the lumen of the artery are determined by the navigation system, which interacts electromagnetically with the catheter tip. These data are processed electronically in conjunction with the ultrasound data to produce real-time images of the artery wall structure in any selected plane. Both the angular and translational (axial) positions of the laser and imaging system are provided to the physician on a continuous basis. The navigation information also permits the physician to return precisely to a previously examined site after completing a plan of attack on a particular lesion.

Figure 2 shows a conceptual detail of the dis-

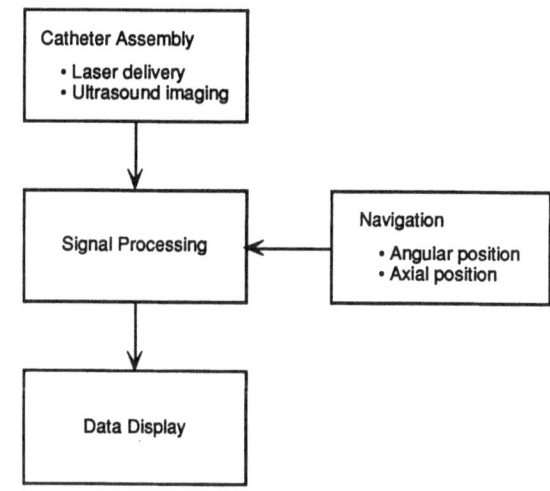

Fig. 1. Major components of the Intra-Sonix laser atherectomy system.

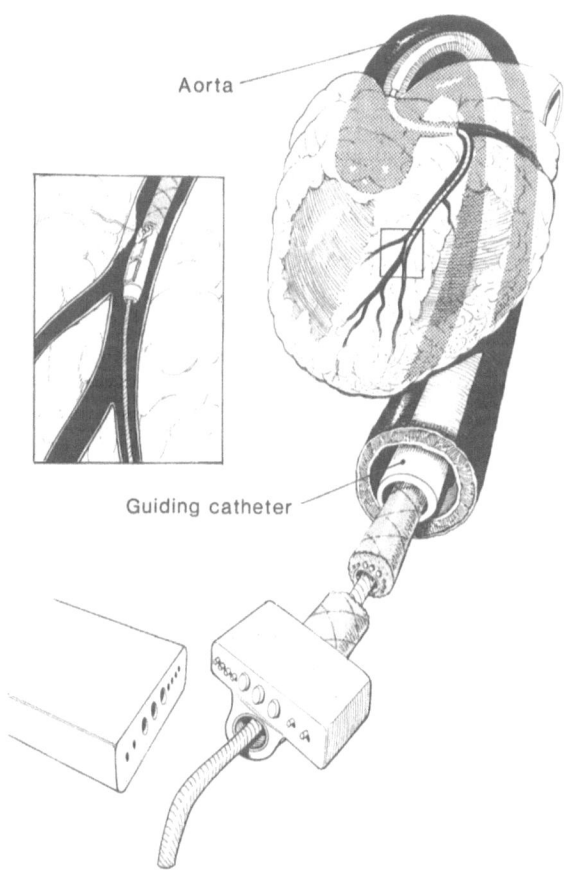

Fig. 2. Artist's conception of the Intra-Sonix catheter assembly, showing position of laser delivery fibers and ultrasound imaging transducer.

posable catheter as it would appear in a coronary artery. It contains a guidewire lumen, fibers for laser beam delivery and the ultrasound imaging device. The distal 5 cm of the catheter is less than 3 F. The laser radiation and ultrasound are codirectional, so the system images the section of the artery toward which the laser is aimed. A photograph of a version of this catheter, designed for imaging tests in small animals, is shown in Fig. 3. It accepts an 0.018 guidewire, as shown.

The radial orientation of the codirectional laser and imaging beams permits ultrasonic depth profiling of the artery tissue structure throughout the thickness of the artery, to allow the physician to determine the level of therapy to be applied and to monitor the depth of plaque removal in progress. The orientation of the optical fibers and ultrasound components enables the catheter to be flexible, while still allowing room for fibers large enough to deliver adequate laser power to the therapy site.

Imaging

An example of an ultrasonic image obtained with the system is shown in Fig. 4. The figure shows radial and transverse B-scan images of an artery section mounted in a plastic tube. The radial image shows a complete cross-section of the artery, while the transverse image shows a section along the arterial axis at a fixed angle. The arrow on the radial image indicates the azimuth of the transverse data, and the arrow on the transverse image indicates the axis position of the radial data.

The imaging system is capable of storing and displaying images at multiple positions along the arterial axis, with real-time updating of these images as the catheter progresses through the vessel lumen. The concept is illustrated in Fig. 5. Several radial images can be pre-set at pre-determined increments for simultaneous display to inform the physician of the tissue structure near the therapy site. More importantly, the image at the current position of the catheter is callable by the physician and displayed in its proper orientation to the pre-set images.

As the catheter moves in the vicinity of the ther-

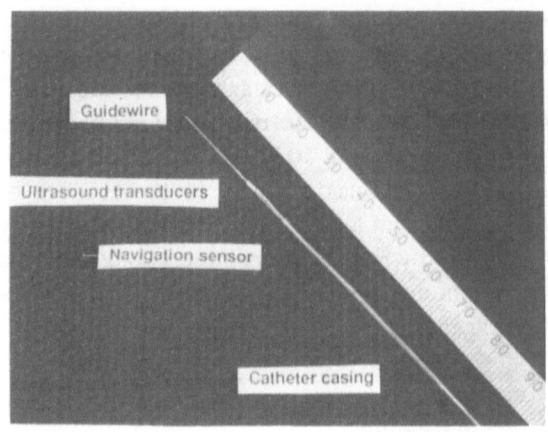

Fig. 3. Experimental catheter assembly.

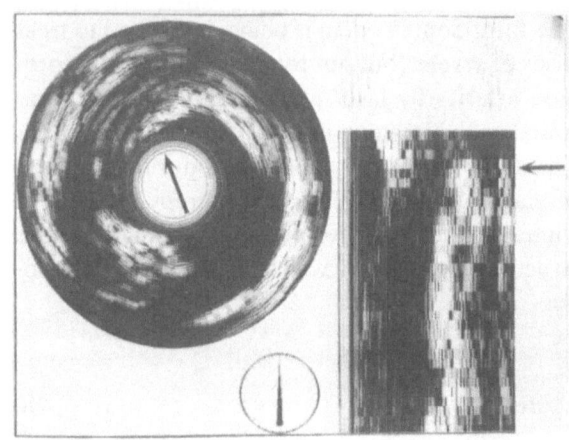

Fig. 4. Radial and transverse (along arterial axis) B-scan images of a tube-mounted artery section.

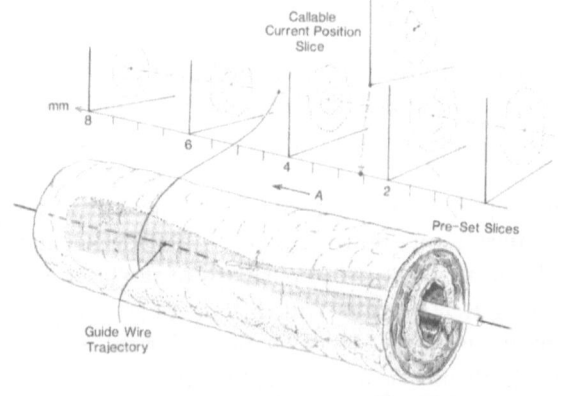

Fig. 5. Three-dimensional display capability of the laser atherectomy system, showing radial images of slices through the artery in their proper orientations.

apy site, the navigation system provides information to allow for image fragments acquired at different points in time to be accumulated into composite images of the artery cross-section at predetermined increments. In this manner, the imaging system constantly updates the images for greater detail at and near the therapy site.

Conclusion

By using some new technical approaches, we have designed and demonstrated the feasibility of an ultrasound-guided transverse laser coronary atherectomy system which adequately meets the ideal requirements for such a system, as described above.

The in vitro results with this system have been sufficiently encouraging that testing in small animals is being undertaken. This program will progress to testing in the canine-human xenograph model over the coming months. Of particular interest in this program will be (a) the ability of the system to correct for motion-induced artifacts in vivo; (b) the ability of the catheter to exhibit in vivo the appropriate 'feel' and controllability required by the interventionalist; and (c) the selection of the most promising laser parameters (wavelength, pulse characteristics, power level, spot size, etc.) for ultimate testing in human clinicals, should such a program be justified.

International Journal of Cardiac Imaging **4**: 159–168, 1989.

Review of intracoronary Doppler catheters

Craig J. Hartley
Baylor College of Medicine, Dept. of Medicine, Sect. of Cardiovascular Sciences, Houston, TX 77030, USA

Abstract

During the last 20 years several types of Doppler catheters have been developed and applied to the measurement of coronary blood flow velocity in man. Validation studies in the laboratory and in animals have shown that these catheters can accurately measure velocity from a small sample volume beside or ahead of the catheter tip. The Doppler transducers have been miniaturized enough (< 1 mm dia) to be mounted on subselective coronary catheters or balloon angioplasty catheters without compromising any of the normal catheter functions. Good quality, high fidelity velocity signals have been recorded from many sites within the coronary circulation of patients during coronary arteriography and balloon angioplasty. Coronary flow reserve measured with Doppler catheters is a physiologic index of the severity of a stenosis which, when carefully measured, can be used for assessing lesions, planning treatment, and evaluating the success of interventions.

Introduction

Although Doppler ultrasound is generally accepted as an important non-invasive modality for assessing blood flow in man, there are several vessels which are inaccessible using standard techniques. Probably the most important of these vessels are the coronary arteries which supply blood to the heart muscle. In addition to being small and relatively deep, coronary arteries are mounted on the moving heart and are surrounded by lung over much of their length. Since cardiac catheterization and balloon angioplasty have become routine procedures in diagnosing and treating coronary artery disease, a catheter-mounted Doppler transducer is an acceptable alternative to a non-invasive probe at least for research applications.

In the past there have been several attempts to construct catheter mounted ultrasonic velocity probes using a variety of techniques. One of the earliest of these was based on the differential transit-time principle [1]. It used two 5 MHz transducers mounted facing each other across a flow-through section 3 cm long near the tip of the 4 mm

diameter catheter [2]. The large physical size of the transducer limited its use to the larger vessels such as the aorta, and it was not practical for use in patients.

Continuous wave Doppler was first applied to catheter mounted transducers by Stegall in 1967 [3]. The transducer consisted of two hemidiscs of 7 to 10 MHz piezoelectric material mounted on the tip of a 7 to 9 French (2.3 to 3.0 mm diameter) standard diagnostic catheter. These were used in several clinical studies of aortic blood flow [4] as well as flows in the cardiac chambers and the great veins. In 1971 Benchimol's group was the first to report the measurement of coronary artery velocity signals in patients using the continuous wave Doppler probe [5]. They were limited by the size of the catheter to measurements in the coronary ostia, and because there was no lumen they were unable to inject contrast agents or to measure pressure at the same site as the flow measurement.

One way to reduce the size of the catheter tip is to eliminate one of the ultrasonic crystals. A continuous wave Doppler can be used with a single crystal by connecting a transformer bridge circuit between the instrument and the catheter. This technique was used by Kalmanson to study flow through the cardiac chambers in dogs [6], and by Reid who made a 3 French (1.0 mm diameter) catheter to record flow signals from within the coronary arteries of dogs [7]. One practical difficulty with the bridge technique is that the impedance of the crystal and its connecting cable must be carefully balanced making the catheter very sensitive to vibration and changes in position.

Another way to utilize a single crystal transducer is to use pulsed rather than continuous wave Doppler. Pulsed Doppler instrumentation was introduced in 1969 by Peronneau [8] and Baker [9]. Since transmission of sound pulses and reception of the resulting echoes are done at different times, the same crystal may be used for both purposes. During the last 15 years several types of catheters based on pulsed Doppler ultrasound have been designed and used to sense coronary blood flow in man.

In 1974 Hartley described a pulsed Doppler flow sensing catheter modified from a Sones coronary catheter [10]. This catheter was used clinically by Cole [11] to measure coronary blood flow velocity in the ostia of native coronary arteries and bypass grafts of patients undergoing diagnostic cardiac catheterization. These catheters demonstrated the concept of measuring vascular reserve as a physiologic index of the severity of coronary lesions [12] and were used in several other research studies [13, 14]. However, the relatively large size (5 French, 1.7 mm) and lack of a steerable guide wire prevented subselective advancement and hindered their widespread use.

Although it was feasible to construct smaller catheters which functioned well [7, 12], the necessary guiding systems for subselective placement were not available until the advent of percutaneous transluminal coronary angioplasty in the 1980's [15]. Angioplasty also provided a need to evaluate the physiologic significance of potentially treatable lesions and to assess physiologic effects of treatment by angioplasty. The first 3 French subselective Doppler catheter to be used in man was described by Wilson in 1985 [16], and the first steerable catheter utilizing a separate guide wire was described by Sibley in 1986 [17]. More recently,

Doppler crystals have been mounted directly on angioplasty balloon catheters eliminating the need for a separate flow sensing catheter [15, 18, 19]. These newer catheters are now available from several commercial sources* and are being extensively evaluated by several institutions. The following paper will review the technical operation, applications, and limitations of currently available pulsed Doppler catheters for evaluating the coronary circulation in man.

Instrumentation

The ultrasonic instruments used with the various coronary velocity catheters are all based on the original design described by Hartley for measuring blood flow with very small transducers [10, 20]. A sketch illustrating the pulsed Doppler principle as applied to catheter-tip transducers is shown in Figure 1. The catheter with the ultrasonic crystal mounted at the tip is positioned in a blood vessel where it lies at some arbitrary angle (θ) to the flow stream. Short bursts of sound are emitted by the crystal which then acts as a receiver for the returning echoes. A range-gate delayed in time from the transmitted burst is used to sample the echoes returning from a specific range or distance. The specific size of this sample volume is determined by the size of the crystal, the length of the transmit burst, the length of the range-gate pulse, and any filtering done within the instrument. The position of the sample volume and its angle to the flow stream are controlled by the range-gate delay and the catheter position. The instrumentation senses the Doppler shifts of the blood cells moving through the sample volume according to the Doppler equation shown at the bottom of Fig. 1. With a stable, fixed position, the angle θ is constant as are the transmitter frequency (f = 20 MHz) and the speed of sound in blood (c = 1,500 m/sec). Thus, the average Doppler shift frequency ($\triangle$f) is directly proportional to

---

* Millar Instruments, Inc., Houston, TX USA: Model DC-101
NuMED, Inc., Hopkinton, NY, USA: Model NuVEL
Schneider, Zürich, Switzerland: Doppler-balloon and Monorail™

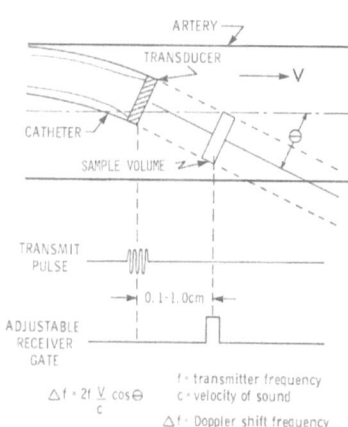

Fig. 1. Sketch of a catheter positioned at an arbitrary angle and location within a blood vessel. The position of the sample volume is determined by the time delay between transmission of the ultrasonic tone burst and the range-gated sampling of the returning echoes. The Doppler equation relating the Doppler shift frequency to the velocity of the blood is shown below.

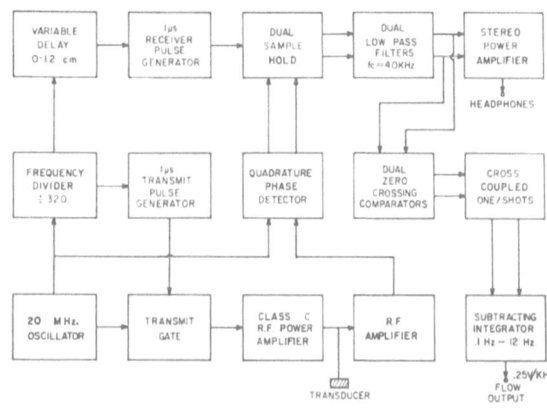

Fig. 2. Block diagram of the directional 20 MHz pulsed Doppler system designed for use with catheter mounted transducers. The PRF of 62.5 KHz allows Doppler shifts up to 31.25 KHz to be sensed at ranges up to 1.2 cm from the catheter tip.

the average velocity (V) within the sample volume. For end-mounted crystals as shown, the angle θ is usually small enough that cosθ = 1, giving V/△f = 3.75 cm/sec/KHz. For side-mounted crystals the angle may be closer to 45 degrees giving V/△f = 5.3 cm/sec/KHz.

Because of the environment in which it operates, a pulsed Doppler system designed specifically for use with small intraluminal transducers will have different characteristics from one designed to operate transcutaneously with larger transducers [10, 20]. The major difference in this design is the relatively high 20 MHz operating frequency which was chosen to maximize the energy received by the <1 mm2 crystal from blood cells. Scattering from red cells is proportional to the fourth power of frequency [21] while the absorption in blood is proportional to frequency raised to the power of 1.2 [22]. In general, the optimal frequency increases with decreasing penetration requirements.

Figure 2 shows a block diagram of the 20 MHz directional pulsed Doppler system specifically designed for use with catheter tip transducers. The 20 MHz oscillator frequency is divided by 320 to generate a pulse repetition frequency (PRF) of 62.5 KHz. A series of 0.4–1.0 usec pulses at the PRF is used to gate 8–20 cycle bursts of the 20 MHz

oscillator signal to the transducer. The transducer converts the electrical signals to ultrasonic tone bursts which propagate into the blood or tissue (Fig. 1) where they are reflected by the various structures encountered (blood cells, vessel walls, etc.). The ultrasonic echoes returning to the transducer are separated in time according to the distance of each reflecting structure. These echo signals are amplified and compared in phase to quadrature signals from the master oscillator. After a variable delay from transmission, the phase signals are sampled (range gated) and these values stored until the sampling interval following the next transmission. The resulting staircase waveforms represent the Doppler shift signal originating at a specific distance from the transducer. The frequency of the Doppler shift is extracted from the two quadrature audio signals by a directional zero crossing counter [23]. The parameters chosen allow velocity components up to 117 cm/sec to be sensed in the direction of the sound beam at distances up to 1.2 cm from the Doppler crystal.

Transducers

Although several catheters have been developed for sensing coronary blood flow in man [5, 11, 15–17, 21], only a few have gained wide acceptance to date. These are the Millar DC-101 [17], the

NuMED NuVEL [16], and the Schneider Mono-rail™ and balloon mounted Doppler sensor [15]. All of these catheters use 20 MHz Doppler crystals, are 1 mm in diameter at the distal tip, have a central lumen for a guide wire, and are designed for subselective use with standard angioplasty introducing systems. There are, however, major differences in how they are configured.

The transducer shown in Fig. 3 (Millar DC-101) is mounted on the 1.0 mm tip of a USCI Rentrop reperfusion catheter originally designed for intra-coronary streptokinase infusion. The crystal has an annular shape with a central hole for the guide wire to pass, and the sound beam extends from the tip in the direction of the catheter. In contrast, the NuMED catheter shown in Fig. 4 has a side mounted rectangular crystal 5 mm from the tip which emits sound at an angle to the catheter. The Schneider balloon Doppler catheters have a tip configuration similar to the Millar DC-101. Except for the Monorail™ catheter, all of these catheters allow intracoronary administration of agents such as vasodilators either through the guiding catheter in the coronary ostia or directly through the lumen of the Doppler catheter.

Validation

Although the original goal in developing flow sensing catheters was to measure true volume flow, these catheters are all designed to sense velocity within a small sample volume remote from the transducer. Several methods have been used to validate the accuracy of the Doppler shift measured by catheter transducers against flow or velocity. These methods include calibration of Doppler shift vs: 1) volume flow through a tube in a flow loop driven by a pump with a calibrated output; 2) volume flow through an artery of an animal measured by timed collection; 3) velocity of a circular trough of liquid rotating at constant speed; 4) velocity of the surface of a rotating turntable; 5) velocity of a loop of suture or magnetic tape driven by a variable speed motor; and 6) velocity of the catheter itself moving through a stationary fluid. The first two methods simulate the situation in a

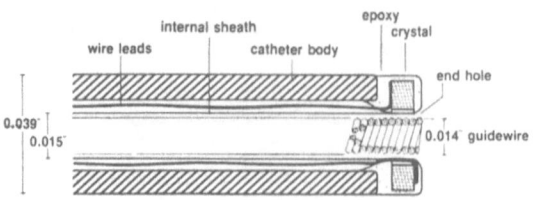

Fig. 3. Cross-sectional drawing of the Millar DC-101 catheter. The ultrasonic crystal is a disc with a central hole providing a lumen for a 0.014″ (0.36 mm) guide wire. The Doppler-tipped balloon catheters have a similar cross-section but with slightly different dimensions.

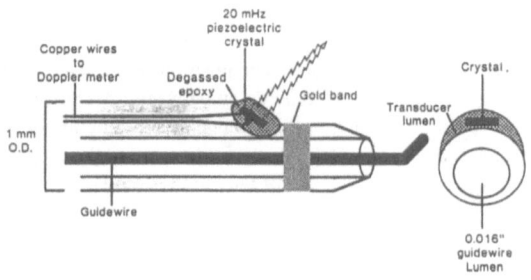

Fig. 4. Drawing of the NuMED NuVEL catheter with the Doppler crystal mounted at an angle on the side 5 mm from the tip.

vessel where the Doppler shift is to be an estimate of volume flow. The last four methods relate the Doppler shift to a known velocity rather than flow. Although each of the methods can be used to evaluate some part of the Doppler-catheter system, none can perfectly simulate all the conditions occurring when a catheter is placed in a coronary artery of a beating heart.

Figure 5 shows a calibration of the Doppler-Sones catheter against volume flow through a canine femoral artery [11]. The curve shows a fairly linear relationship between the Doppler shift and volume flow. Similar linear curves have been generated for the 1 mm Millar [17] and NuMed catheters [16]. The actual slope of the curve depends on the cross-sectional area of the vessel, the angle between the sound beam and the flow axis, the shape of the velocity profile, and the position of the sample volume within the velocity profile. Although the angle is usually close to zero with end-mounted crystals or is known with side-mounted crystals, and the vessel diameter can be estimated

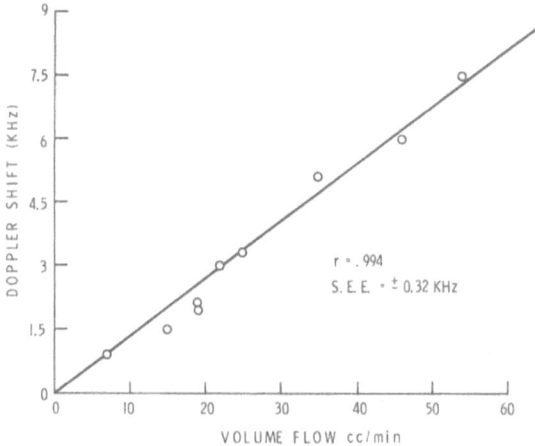

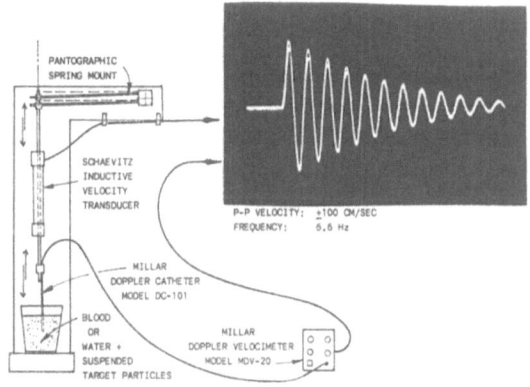

Fig. 5. Calibration of a Doppler-Sones catheter in the femoral artery of a dog relating Doppler Shift frequency in KHz to actual volume flow measured by timed collection in ml/min.

Fig. 6. Drawing of a calibration device incorporating a linear velocity transducer. This system allows direct comparison between actual velocity and the Doppler measured velocity of the catheter moving with respect to the stationary fluid. The oscilloscope tracing in the upper right corner shows the outputs from the linear velocity transducer and the Doppler velocimeter. A Millar DC-101 catheter was used and the range gate was set to 3 mm. The springs were initially deflected, held for several seconds, and then released producing a damped sinusoidal velocity waveform starting at zero. The Doppler signal has the lower amplitude.

by arteriography, the position of the sample volume within the velocity profile is difficult to control or to determine. In addition, the presence of the catheter within the vessel lumen may alter the velocity or the velocity profile at the sample volume site. Thus absolute volume flow cannot be measured reliably with a Doppler catheter system.

Figure 6 shows a calibration device in which the catheter is moved at a known velocity in a stationary fluid [18]. The catheter is connected to a pantographic spring mount which is initially deflected and then released producing a damped sinusoidal vibration. This system provides a linear oscillatory motion with initial peak velocities in excess of 100 cm/sec in each direction. The true instantaneous velocity of the catheter is measured by a linear velocity transducer (LVT) (Schaevitz 6L3 VT-Z) with a 7.6 cm travel. Because the liquid is not moving and the container is large with respect to the catheter, the only change from a flat velocity profile is that introduced by the motion of the catheter itself. The fluid may be whole blood or water with suspended particles. Simultaneous outputs from the LVT and a Millar MDV-20 pulsed Doppler instrument ranged to 3 mm are shown in the upper right corner for the DC-101 catheter. The Doppler output is slightly less than the LVT output at higher velocities because the catheter displaces (pushes and pulls) the fluid around it as it moves back and

forth. In general, however, the agreement is excellent.

Most calibration tests against known velocity show that the Doppler measurement agrees well with the actual velocity within the sample volume. The exception is when there are secondary flows, turbulence, rapid fluctuations in velocity, or a large gradient in velocity within the sample volume. Although turbulence is unlikely to occur in coronary arteries, secondary flow patterns may occur near plaques or branching vessels, disturbances may occur downstream from the catheter, and velocity gradients are large near the vessel walls. High amplitude, low frequency wall motion signals can also cause problems in signal processing if the sample volume is near the wall. In addition, there are many sources of radio frequency (RF) interference in a catheterization laboratory, and if these are picked up by the catheter or Doppler instrument, the velocity measurements may not be valid. Since these phenomena are not constant with velocity or catheter position, any of them could disrupt and invalidate velocity measurements in ways which are difficult to detect in clinical situations and difficult to simulate under controlled laboratory conditions.

Many of these conditions can be detected by listening to the Doppler audio signal. Good quality Doppler signals have a narrow band musical quality and are loud with respect to the normal background hiss. Wall motion causes low frequency 'thumping' sounds. Turbulence or flow disturbances cause harsh, irritating sounds like static on a radio. RF interference usually causes static or tones to be heard. High velocity gradients cause harsh, noisy sounds. Sometimes a slight adjustment in catheter position will correct the problem, but if any of these abnormal sounds can be heard, the resulting velocity measurements should be used with caution.

Clinical applications and results

There are two major applications for Doppler catheters in measuring coronary blood flow velocity: 1) evaluating the physiologic significance of coronary lesions and the results of treatment; and 2) studying the physiology and pathophysiology of coronary blood flow in conscious man. Since Doppler catheters don't measure volume flow and only measure velocity within the sample volume, most of the applications rely on the linearity of the output with volume flow by evaluating the changes in coronary flow in response to an intervention.

It has been shown that for a stenosis to lower resting coronary flow, the reduction in diameter must exceed 85%, but to lower maximal flow during stress or vasodilation only a 35% narrowing is necessary [24]. Thus, resting flow is often normal even with severe stenoses, and to evaluate a lesion it is necessary to increase flow above resting levels with stress or a vasodilator. The amount that flow through the lesion can increase above the resting level is defined as flow reserve which is a physiologic measure of the significance of the lesion [24]. Flow reserve can be estimated as the ratio of peak maximal flow through a lesion during vasodilation (P) to resting flow (R). This ratio (P/R) can be evaluated by measuring velocity with a Doppler catheter immediately proximal to the stenosis during administration of a maximal vasodilator.

The first attempt to evaluate coronary flow reserve in man was reported by Cole in 1977 using a Sones-Doppler catheter to measure proximal coronary velocity and using contrast media as a vasodilator [11]. The response of a non-stenosed human right coronary artery to a 5 cc selective injection of contrast media is shown to the left in Figure 7. For proximal lesions in the right coronary there was a good correlation between P/R and the angiographic severity of the lesion as shown to the right in Fig. 7 [12]. The two open circles in Fig. 7 illustrate shortcomings of both arteriography and the P/R method for evaluating lesions. Point 'A' is a patient with a dilated vessel containing a 75% diameter reduction. The residual lumen was 2 mm, and the normal P/R shows that the lesion was not significant. Point 'B' is a patient with a total occlusion but with several major branches proximal to the lesion. The P/R measurement thus represents flow to the branches and does not evaluate the lesion. In the left main coronary artery, correlations between P/R and lesion severity were poor because the catheter could not be advanced subselectively past the left main into the branch with the lesion.

In the operating room Marcus [25] and White [26] measured flow reserve distal to lesions using a suction Doppler probe and the hyperemic response to a 20 second occlusion as a stress. With these complex lesions, they found a poor correlation between the angiographic appearance of the lesion and P/R. More recent studies by Wilson [27] using the subselective NuMed catheter and papaverine [28] as a vasodilator show a good correlation between P/R and angiographic severity in patients with discrete lesions. Matsumura has shown that P/R measured by Doppler catheter correlates well with clinical severity as measured by exercise tolerance [29]. Thus, when measured properly, flow reserve may be a better indicator of lesion severity than angiography especially for diffuse lesions with complex geometries [26, 30].

The effects of angioplasty on P/R have been studied by several groups. Wilson [31] has shown that angioplasty improves P/R in all patients but returns P/R to normal values (> 3.5 with papaverine) in less than half of the patients. Late (> 4 mo) after angioplasty P/R normalized in all patients in

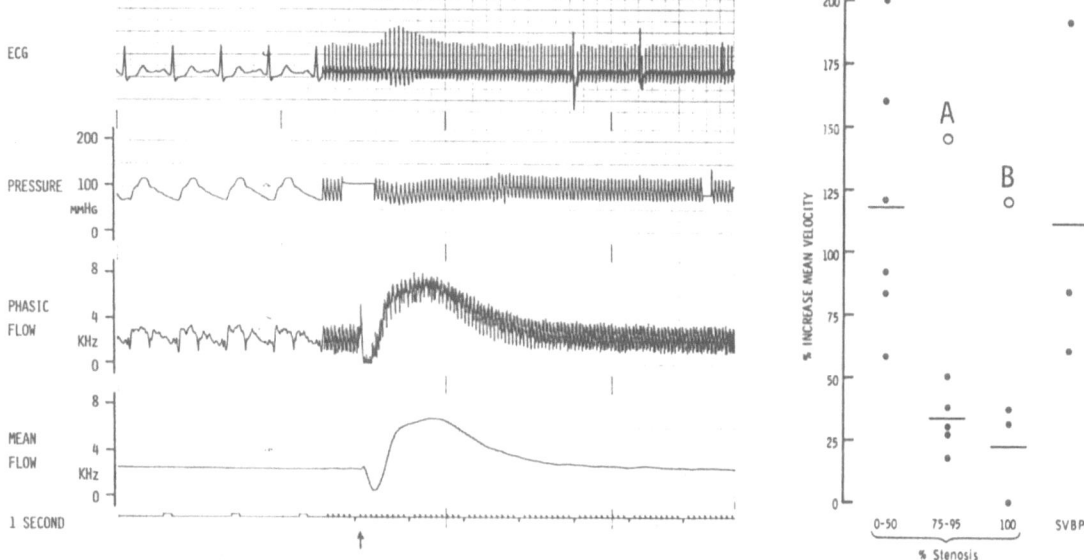

Fig. 7. Example of Doppler signals from the right coronary artery of a patient undergoing diagnostic cardiac catheterization with the Sones-Doppler catheter. Pressure was measured through the lumen of the catheter along with ECG and phasic and mean Doppler signals during an injection of angiographic contrast media (5 cc Hypaque) at the arrow. The peak/resting response to contrast is 2.6 in this patient. To the right is a summary of data from right coronary arteries showing the percent increase in mean velocity = 100(P/R-1) vs percent diameter reduction at the most severe stenosis for 16 patients. Also shown are data from 3 patent saphenous vein bypass grafts (SVBP) to the right coronary artery. The open circles represent 'unusual' cases as explained in the text and were not used in calculating the mean values (bars) at each stenosis.

the absence of restenosis. Similar results have been found by Raymond [32] also using papaverine as a vasodilator and Wainai [33] and Hartley [12] using contrast as a vasodilator. Lesser [34] has used P/R in treatment decisions by deferring angioplasty in stenosed vessels with P/R > 3.5 with papaverine. Late follow-up (20 mo) showed clinical improvement in over 90% of cases while eliminating the restenosis associated with angioplasty.

The effects of coronary bypass grafting on P/R have also been studied by several groups. Cole [11] and Hartley [12] showed that P/R measured with contrast agents using the Doppler-Sones catheter in patent grafts was in the normal range. Wilson [35] has shown similar results in patent grafts with papaverine using the NuMED catheter. Thus, flow reserve as estimated by Doppler catheters 6 to 24 months following successful angioplasty or bypass grafting is normal.

Another potential way to quantify a lesion is to measure the highest velocity at the lesion com-pared to velocity measured proximal to the lesion. If there are no intervening branches, the area-velocity product at the two sites should be equal by continuity. The velocity ratio could then be used to estimate the area reduction [36]. Richards [13] reported detection of left main lesions with the Doppler-Sones catheter by the presence of high velocities. Yeung [37] has validated the method in a tubing model and has noted 20-fold velocity increases in patients when the subselective Doppler catheter is advanced to (but not across) the stenosis. However, this method is not valid if the catheter or guide wire obstructs flow by crossing the lesion, and the difficulty in controlling the sample volume position will make quantification difficult.

Doppler catheters have also been used to study the physiology and pathophysiology of the coronary circulation in man. Vita [38] has shown that intracoronary adenosine increases both coronary flow (322%) and diameter (28%) in a dose-dependent manner. Drexler [39] has shown that normal coronary arteries increase their diameter by 14% in response to the flow increase when papaverine is infused distal to the measurement site. Nabel [40] has shown that this flow-dependent increase is reversed (13% decrease in diameter) in atherosclerotic coronary arteries although nitroglycerine dilated both diseased and normal vessels.

Discussion

Several factors can adversely affect the relationship between coronary flow reserve and P/R as measured with Doppler catheters: 1) the effectiveness of the vasodilating stress or agent; 2) the level of resting flow; 3) the position of the catheter tip, Doppler sensor, and guide wire with respect to the lesion; 4) changes in vessel diameter near the Doppler transducer during the measurement; and 5) alterations in flow or velocity caused by the presence of the Doppler catheter or the guiding catheter.

For measurements of flow reserve to be valid, the intervention must completely dilate the coronary vessels distal to the sensor. Although contrast agents have been used with good success by some investigators [11, 17, 24, 33], others have shown them to be submaximal vasodilators [28, 30]. Intracoronary papaverine has been shown to be a maximal vasodilator with a relatively short action (< 2 min) which is ideal for evaluating flow reserve [28]. The hyperemic response to a brief (20 sec) occlusion has been used to evaluate coronary flow reserve intraoperatively [25], and with the Doppler-tipped balloon catheter, it is now possible to do similar studies in patients before, during, and after angioplasty. However, in chronically stenosed patients, collateral vessels may supply enough flow during occlusion to prevent full dilation [30]. The current vasodilator of choice for evaluating coronary flow reserve is papaverine. In the future adenosine [38] may prove useful due to its even shorter action and lack of effect on the ECG [41] as compared to papaverine which prolongs the Q-T interval.

For P/R to be a good estimate of flow reserve, the arterial bed must be autoregulating and the

resting flow must be normal or below [24]. However, it has been shown that P/R is reduced by pacing [42, 43] and by increases in pressure and cardiac work [44] primarily because resting flow is increased. If possible, P/R should be measured in an angiographically normal vessel to control for differences in resting flow.

Immediately following angioplasty, resting flow may be elevated because the distal bed is not yet autoregulating [31, 32] resulting in low P/R. The time constant of the autoregulatory response to the decrease in proximal resistance may be considerably longer in some patients than the 15 minutes between angioplasty and the subsequent velocity measurements. A better index for angioplasty success may be the ratio of the peak velocity following angioplasty to the resting velocity before [18]. However, this requires that the catheter be placed in precisely the same position for both measurements. Several months (4–49) after successful angioplasty, resting flow and P/R are normal [31].

If there are any branches between the lesion and the Doppler sensor, P/R measurement may represent flow into the branches and not flow through the lesion. Arteriograms must be critically evaluated for visible branches proximal to the lesion, and the Doppler sensor should be advanced beyond major branches if possible.

If the diameter of the coronary artery near the Doppler sensor changes significantly during the measurement, the relationship between Doppler shift and flow will change, and P/R may not represent flow reserve accurately. Adenosine has been shown to increase the diameter of proximal coronary arteries by up to 28% [38], nitroglycerine increases diameter by 17% [39], and elevated flow can increase diameter by 18% [40] or 14% [39]. Thus, it is advisable to pretreat patients with nitroglycerin [27, 28, 31], and to adjust P/R measurements for any changes in cross-sectional area [38, 40] before calculating flow reserve.

It has been shown that the presence of the Doppler catheter in the lumen can affect the velocity downstream from the catheter. Tadaoka [45] measured velocity profiles distal to the tip of a Millar Doppler catheter and found reduced centerline velocity and 'M' shaped profiles as far as 2 cm from the catheter tip. Voyles [46] has shown that with a poor signal-to-noise ratio, velocity can be severely underestimated with standard Doppler signal processing (zero-crossing-counter) compared to spectral analysis. In addition, if the peak frequency in the Doppler spectrum exceeds the Nyquist limit [47] (PRF/2 or 31.25 KHz), these frequencies will be aliased [48], and the velocity will be underestimated. Thus, coronary vascular reserve estimated by the P/R method may be underestimated under poor signal-to-noise conditions, when the sample volume is located in the 'turbulent wake' of the catheter (end-mounted types), when the sample volume is near the wall (side-mounted types), or if there are very high velocities (> 117 cm/sec) within the sample volume.

Conslusions

Pulsed Doppler catheters have been shown to measure instantaneous blood velocity accurately and have been of great value in studying coronary physiology and pathophysiology in man. Coronary flow reserve as estimated by peak-to-resting velocity ratio is a physiologic index which, when used in conjunction with the geometric indices provided by arteriography, is valuable in evaluating and planning the treatment of coronary lesions. However, because of the many uncontrollable factors affecting the measurements, extreme care should be exercised if treatment decisions are to be based on peak-to-resting velocity values.

Acknowledgements

The author would like to thank J.S. Cole and K.L. Richards for their contributions to the development of the Doppler-Sones catheter, M.L. Marcus, R.F. Wilson, and C.W. White for their work in developing the side-mounted Doppler catheter, H.D. Millar and D.H. Sibley for their efforts in developing and evaluating the end-mounted Doppler catheter, and D.W. Baker for his help in designing the 20 MHz pulsed Doppler instrument.

References

1. Plass KG. A new ultrasonic flowmeter for intravascular application. IEEE Trans on Biomed Engrg BME 1964; 11: 154–6.
2. Studer U, Fricke G, Scheu H. Testing of an improved ultrasound flowmeter: technical description and results of testing in vitro. Cardiovasc Res 1970; 4: 380–7.
3. Stegall HF, Stone HL, Bishop VS. A catheter-tip pressure and velocity sensor. Proc 20th ACEMB 1967; 27: 4.
4. Benchimol A, Stegall HF, Maroko PR, Gartlan JL, Brener L. Aortic flow velocity in man during cardiac arrythmias measured with the Doppler catheter-flowmeter system. Am Heart J 1969; 78: 649–59.
5. Benchimol A, Stegall HF, Gartlan JL. New method to measure phasic coronary blood velocity in man. Am Heart J 1971; 81: 93–101.
6. Kalmanson D, Toutain G, Novikoff N. Derai C. Retrograde catheterization of left heart cavities in dogs by means of an orientable directional Doppler catheter-tip flowmeter: a preliminary report. Cardiovasc Res 1972; 6: 309–18.
7. Reid JM, Davis DL, Ricketts HJ, Spencer MP. A new Doppler flowmeter system and its operation with catheter mounted transducers. In: Cardiovascular applications of ultrasound, edited by RS Reneman, New York, American Elsevier, 1974; pp. 183–92.
8. Peronneau PA, Leger F. Doppler ultrasonic pulsed blood flowmeter. Proc 8th ICMBE 1969; 10–11.
9. Baker DW. Pulsed ultrasonic Doppler blood flow sensing. IEEE Trans on Sonics and Ultrasonics 1970; SU-17: 170–85.
10. Hartley CJ, Cole JS. A single-crystal ultrasonic catheter-tip velocity probe. Med Instrum 1974; 8: 241–3.
11. Cole JS, Hartley CJ. The pulsed Doppler coronary catheter: preliminary report of a new technique for measuring rapid changes in coronary artery flow velocity in man. Circulation 1977; 56: 18–25.
12. Hartley CJ, Richards KL, Cole JS. Pulsed Doppler coronary artery catheter transducers. In: SA Altobelli, WF Voyles, ER Greene, eds., Cardiovascular ultrasonic flowmetry. New York: Elsevier, 1985: 279–98.
13. Richards KL, Hartley CJ, Cannon S. Usefulness of Doppler catheters in assessment of coronary artery blood flow. In: MP Spencer, ed., Cardiac Doppler diagnosis. Boston: Martinus Nijhoff 1983: 91–7.
14. Dole WP, Richards KL, Hartley CJ, Alexander GM, Campbell AB, Bishop VS. Diastolic coronary artery pressure-flow velocity relationships in conscious man. Cardiovasc Res 1984; 18: 548–54.
15. Meier B. Coronary angioplasty, Harcourt Brace Jovanovich, New York: 1987: 83–5.
16. Wilson RF, Laughlin DE, Ackell PH, Chilian WM, Holida MD, Hartley CJ, Armstrong ML, Marcus ML, White CW. Transluminal, subselective measurement of coronary artery blood flow velocity and vasodilator reserve in man. Circulation 1985; 72: 82–92.

17. Sibley DH, Millar HD, Hartley CJ, Whitlow PL. Subselective measurement of coronary blood flow velocity using a steerable Doppler catheter. JACC 1986; 8: 1332–40.

18. Hartley CJ, Millar HD. Ultrasonic sensors for measuring coronary blood flow. In: AI West, ed., Microsensors and catheter based imaging technology. Proc. SPIE 1988; 904: 17–22.

19. Juilliere Y, Zijistra F, de Feyter P, Suryapranata H, Serruys PW. Intracoronary blood flow velocity during angioplasty: A functional guide and indicator of the success of dilatation. Arch Mal Coeur 1987; 80: 1725–33.

20. Hartley CJ, Cole JS. A pulsed Doppler system for measuring blood flow in small vessels. J Appl Physiol 1974; 37: 626–9.

21. Reid JM, Sigelmann RA, Nasser MG, Baker DW. The scattering of ultrasound by human blood. Proc 8th ICMBE 1969: 10–7.

22. Carstensen EL, Li K., Schwan HP. Determination of the acoustic properties of blood and its components. J Acoustical Soc Am 1953; 25: 286–9.

23. McLeod FD. A directional Doppler flowmeter. Proc 7th Int Conf on Med and Biol Engr Stockholm 1967: 13–4.

24. Gould LK, Lipscomb K, Hamilton GW. Physiologic basis for assessing critical coronary stenosis: Instantaneous flow response and regional distribution during coronary hyperemia as measures of coronary flow reserve. Am J Cardiol 1974; 33: 87–94.

25. Marcus ML, Wright CB, Doty DB, Eastham CL, Laughlin DE, Krumm P, Fastenow C, Brody MJ. Measurement of coronary velocity and reactive hyperemia in the coronary circulation of humans. Circ Res 1981; 49: 877–91.

26. White CW, Wright CB, Doty DB, Hiratza LF, Eastham CL, Harrison DG, Marcus ML. Does visual interpretation of the coronary arteriogram predict the physiological importance of a coronary stenosis? N Engl J Med 1984; 310: 819–24.

27. Wilson RF, Marcus ML, White CW. Prediction of the physiologic significance of coronary arterial lesions by quantitative lesion geometry in patients with limited coronary artery disease. Circulation 1987; 75: 723–32.

28. Wilson RF, White CW. Intracoronary papaverine: an ideal coronary vasodilator for studies of the coronary circulation in conscious humans. Circulation 1986; 73: 444–51.

29. Matsumura Y, Mishima M, Ohara T, Yamamoto K, Kodama K. Coronary flow reserve by Doppler catheter: Coincident with clinical severity. Circulation 1988; 78 Suppl II: II–256.

30. Marcus ML, Wilson RF, White CW. Methods of measurement of myocardial blood flow in patients: a critical review. Circulation 1987; 76: 245–53.

31. Wilson RF, Johnson MR, Marcus ML, Aylward PE, Skorton DJ, Collins S, White CW. The effect of coronary angioplasty on coronary flow reserve. Circulation 1988; 77: 873–85.

32. Raymond RE, Tuzcu M, Shirey EK, Grigera F, Whitlow PL. Coronary blood flow after angioplasty. Circulation 1988; 78 Suppl II: II–103.

33. Wainai Y, Handa S, Iwanaga S, Kyotani S, Kusuhara M, Abe S, Ohnishi S, Nakamura Y. Coronary flow reserve measured with Doppler catheter in successful angioplasty. Circulation 1988; 78 Suppl II: II–256.

34. Lesser JR, Wilson RF, White CW. Can a physiologic assessment of coronary stenosis avoid unnecessary PTCA? Circulation 1988; 78 Suppl II: II–378.

35. Wilson RF, White CW. Does coronary artery bypass surgery restore normal maximal coronary flow reserve? The effect of diffuse atherosclerosis and focal obstructive lesions. Circulation 1987; 76: 563–71.

36. Freed D, Hartley CJ, Christman KD, Lyman RC, Agris JH, Walker WF. High frequency pulsed Doppler ultrasound: A new tool for microvascular surgery. J Microsurg 1979; 1: 148–53.

37. Yeung AC, Vita JA, Ganz P, Selwin A, Reagan K, Bittl JA. Increased flow velocity in the human coronary stenosis: a simple assessment of stenosis severity. JACC 1989; 13: 131A.

38. Vita Ja, Cox DA, Treasure CB, Fish RD, McLenachan JM, Ganz P, Selwyn AP. Response of human coronary arteries to adenosine. Circulation 1988; 78 Suppl II: II–554.

39. Drexler H, Zeiher A, Wollschlager H, Bonzel T, Just H. Flow-dependent coronary dilation in man. Circulation 1988; 78 Suppl II: II–171.

40. Nabel EG, Ganz P, Selwyn AP. Atherosclerosis impairs flow-mediated dilation in human coronary arteries. Circulation 1988; 78 Suppl II: II–474.

41. Wilson RF, Christensen B, Zimmer S, Laxson D, White CW. Effects of adenosine on the coronary circulation in humans. JACC 1989; 13: 132A.

42. Winniford MD, Rossen JD, Simonetti I, Stark CA. Effect of changes in myocardial metabolism on coronary flow reserve in patients. Circulation 1988; 78 Suppl II: II–256.

43. Wilson RF, McGinn AL, Christensen BV, White CW. Long-term variability on coronary flow reserve: the importance of heart rate. Circulation 1988; 78 Suppl II: II–257.

44. Gould KL, Kirkeeide RL, Buchi ML. Relative coronary flow reserve reflects stenosis severity more accurately than absolute flow reserve during changing aortic pressure and cardiac workload. JACC 1989; 13: 162A.

45. Tadaoka S, Kagiyama M, Ogasawara Y, Tsujioka K, Kajiya F. Accuracy of a 20 MHz Ultrasound Doppler catheter to measure coronary blood flow velocity. Circulation 1988; 78 Suppl II: II–34.

46. Voyles W, Scott B, Teague S, Albert D, Thadani U. Coronary vascular reserve measured using Doppler catheters: Role of Doppler signal processing. Circulation 1988; 78 Suppl II: II–35.

47. Shannon CE. Communication in the presence of noise. Proc IRE 1949; 37: 10–21.

48. Hartley CJ. Resolution of frequency aliases in ultrasonic pulsed Doppler velocimeters. IEEE Trans on Sonics and Ultrasonics SU 1981; 28: 69–75.

International Journal of Cardiac Imaging **4**: 169–176, 1989.
© 1989 *Kluwer Academic Publishers.*

What have we learned about coronary artery disease from high-frequency epicardial echocardiography?

Richard E. Kerber, David D. McPherson, Sara J. Sirna, Alan Ross & Melvin L. Marcus
The Departments of Internal Medicine and Anesthesia University of Iowa College of Medicine Iowa City, Iowa, USA

Abstract

We have used a high frequency epicardial echocardiographic technique to visualize and measure coronary artery lumens and walls in patients undergoing cardiac surgery. A 12 MHz probe (Surgiscan, Biosound Corp.) is sterilized and placed on the exposed epicardial coronary arteries. Transverse cross-sectional views are obtained from the arteries on the anterior surface of the heart: the right coronary artery to the cardiac margin and the left anterior descending coronary artery to the cardiac apex.

Numerous echocardiographic-angiographic-pathological correlations have been obtained from this work. We have validated the echocardiographic lumen and wall measurements by comparing the echo measurements to histological material from pressure-distended coronary arterial segments (from animals and fresh human autopsy specimens). We have shown by comparison with angiography that coronary arteries which appear normal or only minimally diseased by angiograms are often diffusely and severely atherosclerotic. We have also evaluated the shape of atherosclerotic lesions and demonstrated a wide range of lumen shapes (oval, circular, complex) and location within the residual coronary lumen (eccentric vs. concentric). Highly eccentric lesions are characterized by relative preservation of portions of the arterial wall, and this may preserve vasoreactivity of the atherosclerotic vessel. We have also demonstrated remodeling of atherosclerotic lesions: enlargement of the total arterial area (wall plus lumen) as a compensatory mechanism to preserve the arterial lumen in the face of encroaching atherosclerosis.

High frequency epicardial echocardiography offers an accurate, real-time, in-vivo method for the anatomic and functional evaluation of coronary atherosclerosis. This dynamic, in-vivo technique supports and extends information previously obtainable only from pathologic studies. It contributes to our understanding of the pathologic anatomy of coronary artery disease.

Introduction

Coronary atherosclerosis has been traditionally evaluated by two primary methods, necropsy and cineangiography. Although enormous data has been acquired from these approaches, each suffers from specific problems. Patients dying of heart disease of necessity represent a highly selected group: the most severely affected patients. Patients dying of noncardiac diseases could represent an appropriate comparison group, but in such cases less attention is usually paid to the heart and to the coronary arteries. In addition, pathologic examination is done ex-vivo in a nondynamic situation; most important, the arteries are not examined under physiologic distending pressure. Thus, information about arterial wall thickness and lumen area is difficult to interpret.

Coronary cineangiography also is generally performed on a selected group of patients – those with symptoms and preliminary tests suggesting clinically significant coronary disease. The examination affords excellent information on the coronary lumen, but the technique is silhouette based and yields only longitudinal views of the artery. No information is provided on the coronary arterial wall thickness. Moreover, the usual evaluation of such angiograms is based on a measurement of the diameter of the presumed normal vessel and the diameter of the arterial lesion as judged most severe in multiple views. This % diameter stenosis measurement must, therefore, assume that the adjacent wall is truly normal, but this is often not the case [1, 2]. The result of this is that a % diameter stenosis of, for example 50%, could be functionally insignificant in a vessel where the remainder of the artery was truly normal, but highly significant where the remainder of the artery was abnormal, and so the reduction of diameter and area proceeded from an already narrow adjacent artery. This situation is illustrated in Fig. 1.

Computerized three-dimensional reconstruction techniques are available to give an accurate estimate of lumen area. However, these techniques are somewhat tedious and time consuming and do require specialized equipment. Therefore, they are not widely employed in clinical use.

Intraoperative ultrasound evaluation of the coronary arteries: High-frequency epicardial echocardiography

In order to overcome these disadvantages, we have utilized an echocardiographic approach to the intraoperative evaluation of coronary arteries. This technique was pioneered by Sahn et al. [3, 4]. We use a very high frequency device which images at 12 MHz, far higher than the usual 2.25 to 5 MHz frequency devices commonly used for transthoracic echocardiography. This device has a resolution of 0.1–0.2 mm in a phantom, but its depth of field is limited to approximately 2 cm. The echocardiographic probe is sterilized or inserted within a sterile sheath, and placed directly over the exposed epicardial coronary arteries during surgery. To facilitate interpretation of the images, they are obtained prior to the institution of cardiopulmonary bypass; this allows the arteries to be imaged at

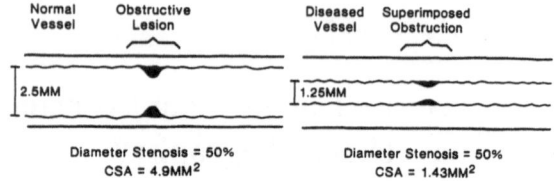

Fig. 1. This diagram illustrates the effects of 50% diameter stenosis in a normal vessel (left panel) and a diffusely diseased vessel (right panel). A 50% diameter stenosis in these two vessel types has a vastly different effect on the cross sectional area (CSA) of the lumen of the vessel at the point of the obstructive lesion. Since the presence or absence of diffuse coronary disease cannot be assessed from visual analysis of coronary angiograms, the functional effect of a coronary stenosis depends on the severity of angiographically undetectable diffuse disease. (Reprinted from Harrison et al. [2], with permission from the American Heart Association, Inc.)

physiological distending pressure. Although cardiac motion sometimes causes technical difficulties in obtaining the images, it is essential to avoid imaging an arrested heart where the arteries would be collapsed, owing to absence of physiologically distending pressure.

The ultrasonic probe, which is manufactured by Biosound, Inc. (Surgiscan), is illustrated in Fig. 2. Owing to the size of the present probe, it is technically difficult to image the arteries on the diaphragmatic or posterior surface of the heart. Thus, at present we image primarily the right coronary artery to the origin of the posterior descending artery, and also the left anterior descending coronary artery.

This approach has major advantages over traditional cineangiographic approaches. We are able to obtain cross sectional as well as longitudinal views of the coronary arteries. This allows determination of true cross sectional lumen area as well as cross-sectional wall thickness, information which is unattainable cineangiographically. The images are real-time images which can be recorded on video tape for subsequent detailed analysis. They are in-vivo and, as noted, obtained under physiologic distending pressure.

Images from our device are shown in Fig. 3. In normal coronary arteries (obtained from patients coming to cardiac surgery for noncoronary indications: congenital heart disease repair, valvular re-

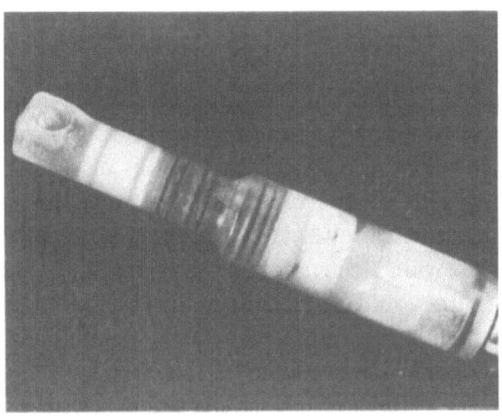

Fig. 2. Illustration of the high frequency echocardiography probe used for our studies. This 12 MHz probe is manufactured by the Biosound Corp. (Surgiscan). Reproduced from McPherson and Kerber, 1986 Echocardiography 3: 371–381, by permission.

pair or placement) the arterial lumen can be well imaged and is free of atherosclerosis. The visualized arterial wall of the ultrasonic recordings is composed of the arterial intima, media and surrounding dense adventitia. The border between dense adventitia and surrounding loose adventitia is generally imaged as a cleavage plane on the ultrasonic recordings. Atherosclerosis is seen as protruding or encircling plaques within the arterial lumen and a corresponding reduction in residual lumen area (Fig. 3).

In order to make quantitative measurements of these lesions, we have undertaken a series of validating studies [5]. Histologic comparisons of lumen area and wall thickness obtained by high frequency echo have been made to similar measurements from histologic specimens. Both echo and histology measurements were made on arteries distended to equivalent pressure. We used arteries from larger animals: sheep, calves and pigs, which closely approximate human coronary arterial size. Excellent correlations were obtained. We then performed similar validating measurements on normal and atherosclerotic human arteries obtained freshly postmortem; again good correspondence with the measurements were shown. These correlations are shown in Fig. 4. Finally, we used a dynamic technique, sonomicrometers, to compare to in-vivo animal arterial diameter measurements and once again a high level of correlation was achieved (Fig. 5).

Echocardiographic-angiographic correlations using high frequency echo

Pathological studies for many years have suggested that coronary atherosclerosis is generally more extensive than coronary angiography reveals [6]. We wanted to demonstrate this using the high frequen-

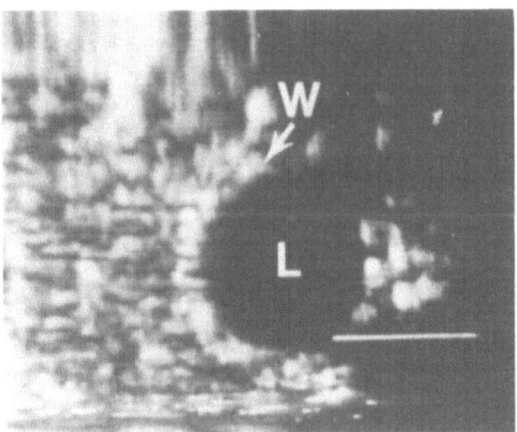

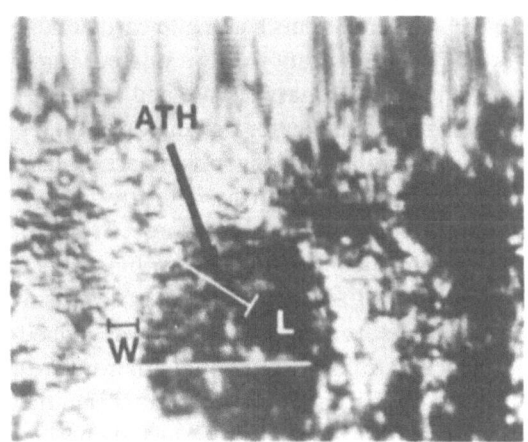

Fig. 3. High frequency echocardiographic stop-frame video images of coronary arteries in cross section from a patient having no angiographic evidence of coronary arterial disease (left panel) and from a patient having severe coronary arterial disease (right panel). W = wall. L = lumen. ATH = atherosclerosis. Reference bar for both studies is 3 mm in length. Reproduced from McPherson and Kerber, (1986) Echocardiography 3: 371–381, by permission.

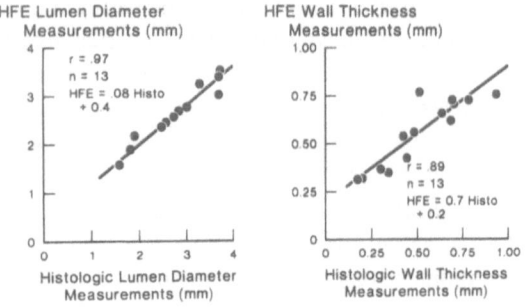

Fig. 4. Comparison of human coronary arterial diameters by histology vs. the high frequency echocardiographic technique. Reproduced from McPherson et al. [5], by permission.

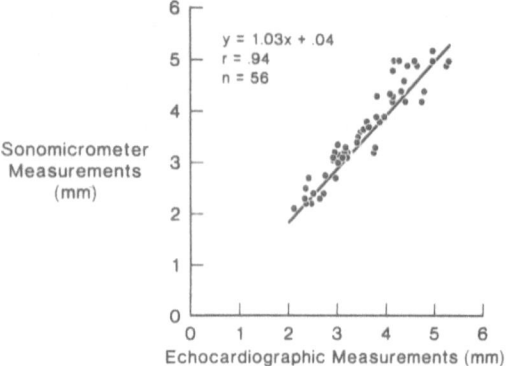

Fig. 5. Comparison of animal coronary arterial diameters by the high frequency echocardiographic technique and by sonomicrometers. Reproduced from McPherson et al. [5], by permission.

cy echo technique. Patients coming to cardiac surgery for numerous indications were studied; some of the patients had coronary disease and were specifically being operated on for that disease, whereas others had valvular or congenital heart disease with no coronary atherosclerosis. The arterial segments were divided into three groups: Group I: images were obtained from patients with no angiographic evidence of any coronary atherosclerosis, Group II: images from an area which was judged angiographically to have substantial atherosclerosis, and Group III: patients who had substantial atherosclerosis elsewhere in the artery being imaged, but little or no disease in the area on which the echocardiographic probe was placed. We calculated lumen diameter to wall thickness ratios for these three groups. In a normal artery with a large

lumen and a thin wall (absence of coronary atherosclerosis) the ratio would be high and this was found, as was expected in Group I. In the patients from Group II where the arterial segments being imaged had angiographically obvious disease, the ratio would be expected to be lower and this was also what was found. However, in the Group III patients where the angiographic data suggested that there would be little or no disease and therefore a high lumen diameter to wall thickness ratio, many of the patients could be shown to have a low ratio (1). This strongly suggested that coronary atherosclerosis was present but was not being demonstrated angiographically. Figure 6 shows the lumen diameter/wall thickness ratios from the different groups, while Fig. 7 shows an example of severe echo-demonstrated atherosclerosis in an artery which appears only mildly diseased by angiography.

Another area of investigation using the high frequency epicardial echo technique has concentrated on the shapes of atherosclerotic lesions. It has been well shown by pathologic studies [7, 8, 9] that the lumens of coronary atheroma lesions show considerable variation in their shape (round, oval, com-

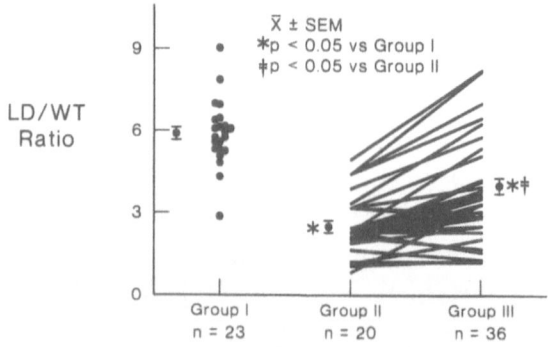

Fig. 6. Ratios of lumen diameter to wall thickness in patients who have no coronary disease (Group I), angiographic stenosis in the area being imaged by high frequency echo (Group II) and angiographic stenosis remote from the area being imaged (Group III). For comparative purposes, connected points indicate segments in both groups II and III from individual patients (see text). Note the abnormal (low) lumen diameter-wall thickness ratio of many arteries in Group III; this indicates that diffuse atherosclerosis can be demonstrated by high frequency echo in vessels which appear relatively normal by angiography. Reproduced from McPherson et al. [1], by permission.

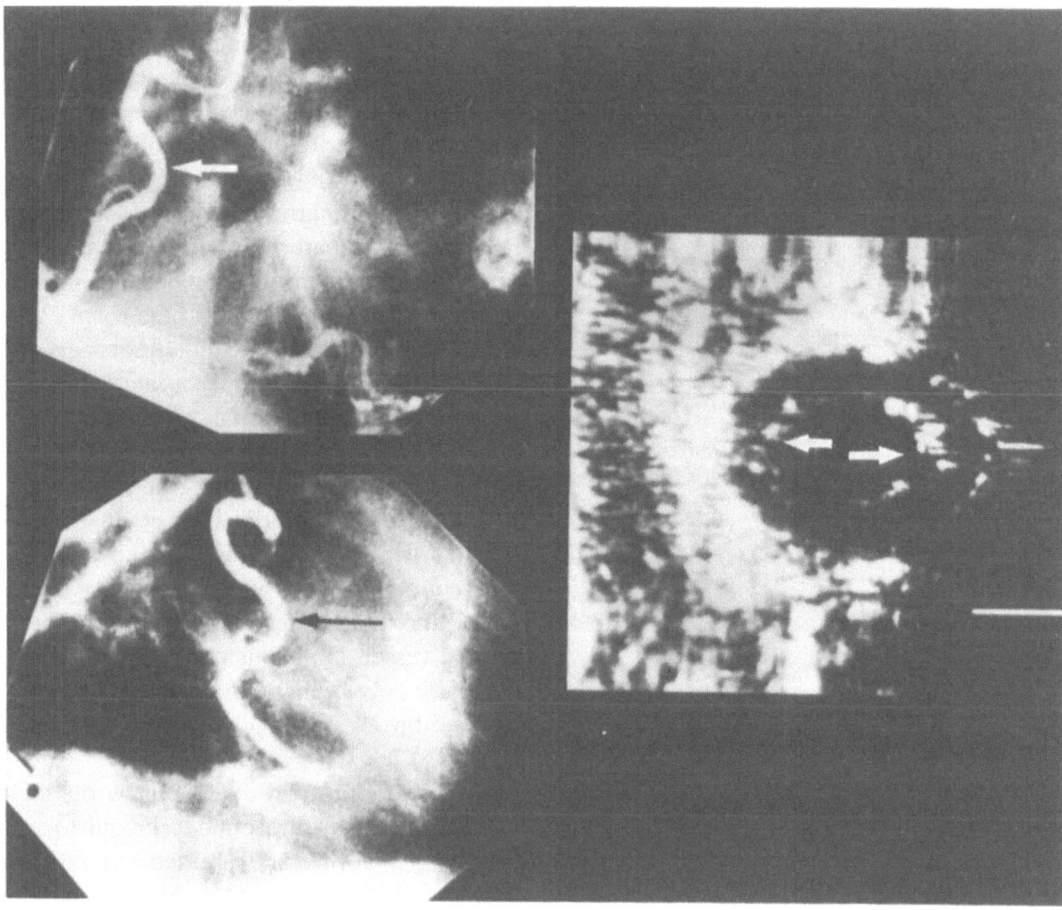

Fig. 7. An example of severe atherosclerosis demonstrated by high frequency echo (right panel), in a patient whose angiogram demonstrates only minimal disease (arrows, left panel). Reproduced from McPherson et al. [1], by permission.

plex) and in their location within the original lumen, that is eccentric-vs. concentric. These studies have recently been reviewed by Waller [10]. Examples of the variable shapes of coronary lesions, shown diagramatically, are provided in Fig. 8. A markedly eccentric location may, of course, result in some portion of the original vessel's circumference being spared from atherosclerotic involvement. Again, because of the angiographic restriction to longitudinal imaging, there has been no readily available in-vivo technique to verify this. Using high frequency epicardial ultrasound, we have conducted a detailed analysis of the shape of atherosclerotic regions [11]. We found that complex shapes occur relatively infrequently (only 3 of the 31 lesions we visualized had complex shapes).

We defined 'circular' lumens as those with a major to minor lesion diameter equal to or less than 1.5 : 1, and 'oval' lesions as those with a diameter greater than 1.5 : 1. Oval lesions occurred in 13 of the 31 lesions; circular lesions in 15. Normal arterial wall thickness is less than 0.7 mm. Portions of the arterial wall were within this normal range in 16 of the 31 lesions we studied. An algorithm to determine eccentricity of the residual lumen within the original lumen was derived; 7 of the 31 residual lumens were eccentrically placed within the original lumen.

174

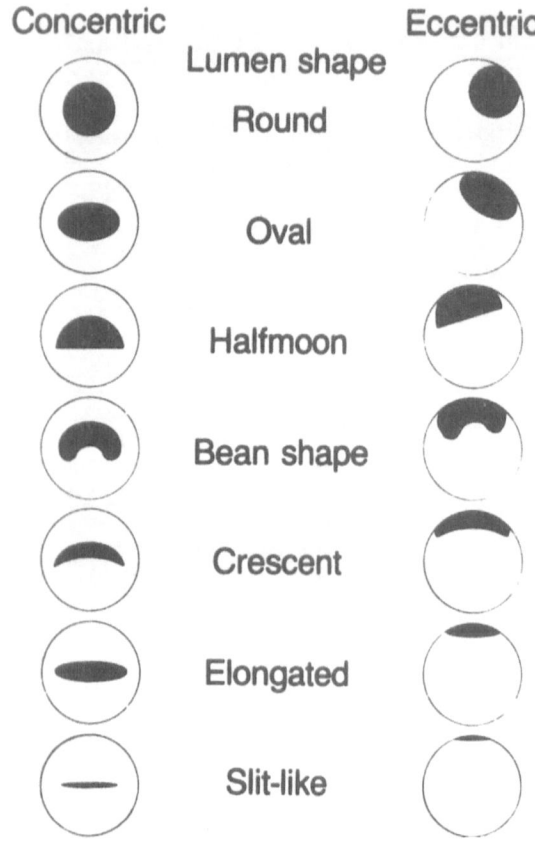

Concentric Eccentric

Lumen shape
Round

Oval

Halfmoon

Bean shape

Crescent

Elongated

Slit-like

Fig. 8. Diagram showing various luminal configurations of eccentric and concentric coronary atherosclerotic plaques. Reproduced from Waller [10]. Copyrighted and reprinted with the permission of Clinical Cardiology/FACM, Inc., The JBI Building, Box 832, Mahwah, N.J. 07438, USA.

Remodeling of atherosclerotic coronary arteries

As coronary atherosclerosis develops, alterations of coronary arterial size and shape have been noted by both pathologic examination of necropsy specimens and by experimental animal studies. Atherosclerotic primates develop enlargement of intimal area (atheroma), but at the same time the lumen area is maintained. This implies that the total size of the artery enlarges [12]. This process, which we have termed arterial remodeling, has been supported by pathologic studies by Glagov et al. [13] which showed, in left main coronary arteries of patients coming to necropsy, that lumen area was maintained despite encroaching atherosclerosis.

The mechanism of such maintenance was enlargement of the outer circumference of the artery. These in-vitro and in-vivo studies have recently been supported by studies of atherosclerotic human carotid arteries by Blankenhorn and co-workers [14] who showed that in longitudinal ultrasound images of carotid arteries diseased segments had a larger outer diameter. This arterial remodeling appears to be an important compensating mechanism by which the hydraulic effect of coronary atherosclerosis is minimized. We studied coronary arteries of patients with and without coronary atherosclerosis and showed in normal vessels that both the lumen area and outer circumference (total arterial area) of arteries diminishes when one compares mid to proximal arterial images. In contrast, in patients with coronary disease, the total arterial area *enlarges* rather than diminishes, when comparing the images from lesions to more proximal normal vessels [15]. This remodeling process precedes the development of angiographic collaterals and may be related to the severity of lumen narrowing [16].

We are presently evaluating using the high frequency epicardial ultrasound technique to evaluate the ability of normal and diseased coronary arteries to respond to a vasodilator, nitroglycerin, and a vasoconstrictor, phenylephrine, when administered intravenously during cardiac surgery. These ongoing studies have demonstrated that even atherosclerotic arteries are able to vasodilate and vasoconstrict, although the degree of such vasodilation and vasoconstriction may be related to the severity of the atherosclerosis [17]. An important consideration here may be the extent of the uninvolved wall, which was alluded to earlier in our discussion of the shape and position of atherosclerotic lesions; an eccentric location of a coronary lesion may result in considerable preservation of normal arterial circumference and this uninvolved segment of the artery may be highly vasoreactive and may also be implicated in the development of coronary vasospasm [10].

Saphenous vein of internal mammary artery graft anastomoses to native coronary vessels have been studied by our high frequency echo technique [18]. We have learned that in general most anastomoses are accomplished with a high degree of precision and adequacy. However, occasionally technical difficulties cause the anastomoses to be unsuitable. This may result in poor flow. Measurements of flow through vein grafts using electromagnetic flow probes have been made, but a low flow state could be either due to a poor anastomosis or to disease downstream. The high frequency echo technique allows differentiation between the two. If a poor anastomosis is demonstrated, an immediate revision of the anastomotic site is feasible. One point which seems to be emerging from these ongoing studies is that side-to-side anastomoses tend to be smaller than end-to-side anastomoses [18]. Whether the difference is clinically significant has not yet been clearly established.

Although saphenous vein graft diameters are larger than internal mammary artery diameters, a comparative study of the anatomoses from these two grafts showed no significant difference between the two [19]. This is important since the long term patency rate of internal mammary arteries is probably higher than saphenous vein grafts; if the small size of the internal mammaries were to result in smaller anastomosis this would be unfavorable. Our echo studies suggest that this is not the case.

High frequency echo technique has also contributed information to coronary arterial anatomy and physiology when combined with other techniques. We have compared high frequency echo images to videodensitometric integrated optical density obtained from orthogonal cineangiographic projections. We found that optical densities from LAO vs. RAO views were nearly identical despite differences in shape, i.e. circular vs. oval/complex. Thus, as long as the vascular segment of interest was parallel to the image intensifier, we were able to show that the results of videodensitometry were not influenced by angiographic projection and lumen shape [20]. This is important in understanding the potential of videodensitometry which is a nongeometric method of assessing coronary lumen area from angiograms.

We have also correlated high frequency echo techniques with measurements of coronary flow reserve assessed by intraoperative Doppler miniaturized suction probes. A brief period of atraumat-ic coronary occlusion by the surgeon results in reactive hyperemia upon reperfusion after 20 seconds of occlusion. If disease upstream is present, this reactive hyperemic response is impaired and this is an important clue to the functional significance of the lesions. We were able to demonstrate significant differences between reactive hyperemia in a group of coronary vessels which were considered to be normal by high frequency echo vs. a group in which high frequency echo showed atherosclerosis [21]. Thus, there was a correspondence between anatomic abnormalities seen by high frequency echo and functional abnormality seen by the intraoperative Doppler flow measurements. This supports the accuracy of the Doppler flow measurements as predictors of functionally significant lesions.

What is the future of this technique? Smaller high frequency echo probes should allow more extensive intraoperative examination of the entire epicardial coronary tree and more detailed visualization of atherosclerotic lesions. Tissue characterization techniques, analyzing ultrasonic backscatter and/or tissue texture, obtained from intra-operative high frequency images, hold considerable potential for distinguishing between blood, lumen and arterial wall [22].

In conclusion, high frequency epicardial echocardiography has yielded valuable new information concerning the pathologic anatomy and functional significance of coronary atherosclerosis. At the same time it appears a useful clinical tool for evaluating the presence and extent of atherosclerosis, and assisting in surgical approaches to coronary disease.

References

1. McPherson DD, Hiratzka LF, Lamberth WC, Brandt B, Hunt M, Kieso RA, Marcus ML, Kerber RE. Delineation of the extent of coronary atherosclerosis by high frequency epicardial echocardiography. New Engl J Med 1987; 316: 304–309.
2. Harrison DG, White CW, Hiratzka LF, Doty DB, Barnes DH, Eastham CL, Marcus ML. The value of lesion cross-sectional area determined by quantitative coronary angiography in assessing the physiologic significance of proximal

left anterior descending coronary arterial stenosis. Circulation 1984; 69: 1111–1119.

3. Sahn DJ, Barrett-Boyes BG, Graham K, Kerr A, Roach A, Hill D, Brandt PWT, Copeland JG, Mammana R, Tempkin LP, Glenn W. Ultrasonic imaging of the coronary arteries in open chest humans: Evaluation of atherosclerotic lesions during cardiac surgery. Circulation 1982; 66: 1034–1044.

4. Sahn DJ, Copeland JG, Tempkin LP, Wirt DP, Mammana R, Glenn W. Anatomic-ultrasonic correlations for intraoperative open chest imaging of coronary artery atherosclerotic lesions in human beings. J Am Coll Cardiol 1984; 3: 1169–1177.

5. McPherson DD, Armstrong M, Rose E, Kieso RA, Megan M, Hunt M, Hite P, Marcus ML, Kerber RE. High frequency epicardial echocardiography for coronary artery evaluation: in-vitro and in-vivo validation of arterial lumen and wall thickness measurements. J Am Coll Cardiol 1986; 8: 600–606.

6. Arnett EN, Isner JN, Redwood DR, Kent KM, Baker WP, Ackerstein H, Roberts WC. Coronary artery narrowing in coronary heart disease: comparison of cineangiographic and necropsy findings. Ann Int Med 1979; 91: 350–356.

7. Vlodaver Z, Edwards JE. Pathology of coronary atherosclerosis. Prog Cardiovasc Dis 1971; 14: 156–174.

8. Freudenberg H, Lichtlen PR. Das Normale Wandsegment bei Koronarstenosen – eine postmortale Studi. Z Kardiol 1981; 70: 863–869.

9. Barode G. Diseases of the coronary arteries, in MD Silver (Ed.), Cardiovascular Pathology, Churchill, Livingstone, New York 1983, pp. 341–342.

10. Waller BF. The eccentric coronary atherosclerotic plaque: Morphologic observations and clinical relevance. Clin Cardiol 1989; 12: 14–20.

11. McPherson DD, Collins SC, Hunt M, Hiratzka L, Marcus M, Kerber RE. Ultrasonic intraoperative evaluation of coronary lesions. J Am Coll Cardiol 1986; 7,1A (Abst).

12. Armstrong ML, Heistad DD, Marcus ML, Megan MB, Piegors DJ. Structural and hemodynamic responses of peripheral arteries of Macque monkeys to atherogenic diet. Arteriosclerosis 1985; 5: 336–346.

13. Glagov S, Weisenberg E, Zarins CK, et al. Compensatory enlargement of human atherosclerotic coronary arteries. New Engl J Med 1987; 316: 1371–1375.

14. Barth JD, Blankenhorn DH, Wickham E, Lai JY, Chin HP, Selze RH. Quantitative ultrasound pulsation study in human carotid artery disease. Arteriosclerosis 1988; 8: 778–781.

15. McPherson DD, Hunt M, Hiratzka LF, Brandt B, Lamberth WC, Marcus ML, Kerber RE. Coronary atherosclerosis causes remodeling of arterial geometry: Demonstrated by high frequency epicardial echocardiography. Circulation 1986; 74: II–468 (Abst).

16. McPherson DD, Johnson MR, Kerber RE. Is remodeling of atherosclerotic arteries related to the severity of luminal narrowing? Evaluation by intraoperative high frequency epicardial echocardiography. Circulation 1988; 78: II–418 (Abst).

17. McPherson DD, Ross AF, Moyers JR, Hiratzka LF, Brandt B, Hunt M, Kerber RE. Can atherosclerotic coronary arteries vasodilate? An intraoperative high frequency epicardial echocardiographic study. Circulation 1986; 74: II–468.

18. Hiratzka LF, McPherson DD, Lamberth WC, Brandt B, Armstrong ML, Schroder E, Hunt M, Kieso RA, Megan MD, Thompkins PK, Marcus ML, Kerber RE. Intraoperative evaluation of coronary artery bypass graft anastomosis with high frequency epicardial echocardiography: Experimental validation and initial patient studies. Circulation 1986; 73: 1199–1205.

19. Sirna SJ, McPherson DD, Meng R, Hiratzka L, Ross A, Kerber RE. Intraoperative high frequency echo comparison of internal mammary artery vs. saphenous vein to native coronary anastomosis. Circulation 1988; 78(Suppl II): II–419 (Abst).

20. Johnson MR, McPherson DD, Fleagle SR, Hunt M, Hiratzka LF, Kerber RE, Marcus ML, Collins SM, Skorton DJ. Videodensitometric analysis of human coronary artery stenosis: Validation in-vivo by intraoperative high frequency epicardial echocardiography. Circulation 1988; 77: 328–336.

21. McPherson DD, Hiratzka LF, Brandt B, Lamberth WC, Hunt M, Hartman J, Clothier J, Eastham C, Kerber RE. Relationship of echo-demonstrated coronary atherosclerosis to reactive hyperemia. Circulation 1986; 74: II–85 (Abst).

22. McPherson DD, Sirna SJ, Haugen JA, Fleagle SR, Thorpe LJ, MacIsaac HC, Rewcastle NB, Armstrong ML, Burns TL, Meng RL, Hiratzka LF, Collins SM, Kerber RE, Skorton DJ. Acoustic properties of normal and atherosclerotic human coronary arteries: in-vitro and in-vivo comparisons. Circulation 1987; 76: IV–43 (Abst).

International Journal of Cardiac Imaging **4**: 177–185, 1989.
© 1989 *Kluwer Academic Publishers.*

Analysis of backscattered ultrasound from normal and diseased arterial wall

David T. Linker, Paul G. Yock[1], Åge Grønningsæther, Erling Johansen & Bjørn A.J. Angelsen
Department of Biomedical Engineering and Division of Cardiology, Regional Hospital, University of Trondheim, N-7006 Trondheim, Norway; [1] Division of Cardiology, M-1186, University of California, San Francisco, California 94143, USA

Abstract

Intra-arterial ultrasonic imaging has several features which affect the feasibility of clinical tissue characterization when compared with trans-thoracic ultrasound. The short distance from transducer to tissue, fluid path, high frequencies, and special characteristics of the tissues of interest all contribute to making practical tissue characterization by measurement of the backscattered signal more probable in intra-arterial imaging. The properties of backscattered ultrasound, and methods of characterizing such signals, are discussed with special reference to intra-arterial applications.

Introduction

The alteration of the backscattered ultrasound signal produced by various mycardial disease states is well known [1–3], and is related to the value and distribution of acoustic properties within the tissue. It has not been possible to use these alterations to uniquely identify pathology because the changes produced are non-specific.

Intra-arterial ultrasound imaging [4, 5] is a new technique using ultrasound to image the structure and content of atheroma in areas of stenosis. The proximity of the structures of interest, the fluid-filled acoustic path, and the resulting high frequencies used allow greater opportunities for tissue characterization in this setting than in traditional trans-thoracic echocardiography. This article is intended as an overview of the issues involved, with special reference to potential advantages and disadvantages of intra-arterial ultrasound imaging.

Properties of backscattered ultrasound

In general, we can categorize the standard methods of ultrasonic tissue characterization based on the backscattered signal as being based on backscattered amplitude or power, the frequency dependency of the backscatter, the frequency dependency of attenuation, and the pattern of the backscatter. Transmission characteristics, such as absolute attenuation and velocity, are difficult to measure in the backscattered signal.

Resolution limits

Backscattering of ultrasound occurs because the sound encounters an interface between areas of differing acoustic properties. The properties which can affect backscatter are the mass density, compressibility, and viscosity. Ideally, the backscattered ultrasound signal would be uniquely associated with the distribution of acoustic properties in the tissue of interest. Unfortunately, the characteristics of the received backscattered ultrasonic signal are the result of many factors in addition to the tissue properties, and different tissue structures can result in similar signals. This is due, in large part, to the averaging effects of the transmitted pulse.

Pulse length and frequency. As a simplifying approximation, we can ignore attenuation and multiple scattering effects. In this case, the backscattered signal is generated solely by the interaction of the transmitted pulse and the interfaces between areas of differing acoustic properties within the tissue. The result is a spatial weighted average, or convolution, dependent on the three dimensional pulse shape and frequency. Features significantly smaller than one half wavelength are averaged and therefore cannot be resolved. Because the sound travels both out to the structures and back to the transducer, there is a factor of one half in the radial direction. The maximum length of the averaging is therefore equal to half the pulse length in the radial direction, and the pulse width in the lateral directions. As a result, structures larger than half the pulse length are clearly resolved in the radial direction, and structures larger than pulse width are readily resolved in the lateral directions. Structures that are of a size between these two limits result in a more complex interaction.

A significant complicating factor is that the pulse shape varies as a function of depth, and is usually affected by side lobes, the effects of refraction, and multiple scattering. The maximum resolution limits mentioned above are theoretical, and then only achieved at the geometric focus of the transducer.

Resolution-frequency relationship. If we calculate these limits for typical trans-thoracic ultrasound, based on a frequency of 3.5 MHz, and a speed of sound of 1560 m/sec, one wavelength is 0.44 mm in length, so the lower limit is 0.22 mm, while the upper limit would be 1.1 mm, based on a pulse length of 5 cycles. If we increase the frequency to 20 MHz, which is common for intra-arterial imaging, one wavelength is 0.078 mm, so that the corresponding limits are 0.039 mm to 0.195 mm.

If the scale of the variation in acoustic properties is significantly smaller than the wavelength, the information we can extract is limited to the backscattered power. This is because the pattern of backscatter will be determined primarily by the response characteristics of the transducer. For variations larger than the pulse length, we can use texture measures or analysis of the autocorrelation function, while variations of intermediate size can produce more complex effects.

Backscattered power

Backscattered power is the total energy per time of the backscattered signal, integrated over all frequencies. The value is usually converted to a ratio, by comparing it to the power reflected from a steel surface, and this ratio is normally reported on a logarithmic scale, in decibels (dB). Backscattered power is affected by both the absolute acoustic properties and their spatial frequency in the tissue. The difference between the acoustic properties of a tissue and its surroundings results in a reflected signal, and there is a signal from each such interface. As a result, the absolute acoustic properties, the spatial frequency of the variation of properties, and the spatial density of interfaces all contribute to the backscattered power [6].

Frequency dependency of backscatter

The backscattered power from a dense collection of scatterers or acoustic interfaces is a function of the frequency and the size of the scatterers or variation in acoustic properties. As the frequency increases, so does the reflection coefficient. The rate at which the backscatter increases with frequency is dependent on the size of the scatterers.

Rayleigh scattering. If the size of the scatterers is significantly smaller than the wavelength, the backscattered power will increase as the fourth power of the frequency increase [7]. This means that a doubling in frequency will result in a sixteenfold increase in the backscattered power.

Larger discrete scatterers. If the size of the scatterers is significantly larger that the wavelength, there will be interference between the backscattered signal from differing points on the surface, and this will reduce to total power. As a result, the backscattered energy will increase roughly as the second power of the increase in frequency. This means that

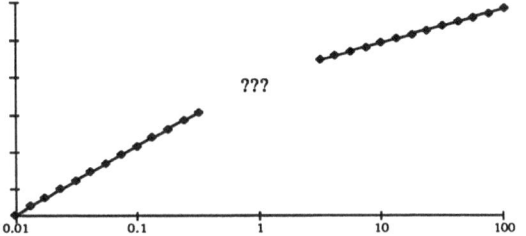

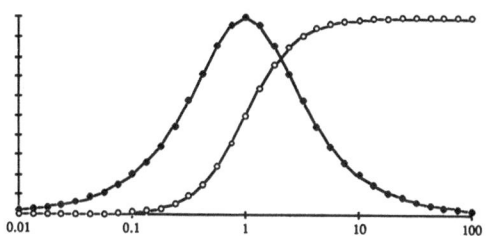

Fig. 1. Theoretical plot of scattering coefficient as a function of frequency. The horizontal axis is frequency, while the vertical axis is the energy scattering coefficient. Both scales are logarithmic, but the value '1' on the frequency scale is when the wavelength is equal to the mean size of the scatterers. The portion on the right is a simplified representation of scattering when the wavelength is much smaller than the objects or scale of variation in acoustic properties, while the portion on the left represent the relationship when the wavelength is larger than the scatterers or acoustic variations (Rayleigh scattering). The slope is equal to the exponent of the frequency dependency. It is 4 in the left-hand portion, and a lesser value in the middle and right hand portions. When the size is intermediate, the relationship is more complex.

Fig. 2. Relationship between attenuation and frequency. The horizontal axis is frequency, normalized to the frequency of maximum attenuation per wavelength, on a logarithmic scale. The open circles represent attenuation as a function of frequency, while the closed circles represent attenuation as a function of wavelength [10].

a doubling in frequency will result in four times the backscattered energy.

Frequency dependency of attenuation

Attenuation is due to both scattering and absorption of the acoustic energy. As would be expected, it also is dependent on frequency, but its measurement is difficult in backscattered signals [8]. This is due primarily to the frequency dependent backscatter form the tissue at maximum depth, which will also contribute to the frequency dependency. It may be possible to compensate for this using estimation techniques [9].

Attenuation is normally expressed as a function of distance, but in the analysis of frequency dependence, it can be useful to express it as a function of distance in wavelengths. The theoretical curves in Fig. 2 are based on scattering from droplets in air.

As can be seen in Fig. 2, the slope of the relationship is markedly variable, and dependent on how close we are to the 'relaxation frequency', or frequency of maximum attenuation. If we allow for

more complex structures than spheres, the resulting attenuation-frequency functions also become more complex [11].

Pattern of backscatter

First order statistics. If we consider the factors which might affect the variation in backscatter from one area to another with similar characteristics, we can easily think of two. The first is the statistical variability, since the power of the backscatter is a function of the number of scatterers per volume, which is presumably Poisson distributed. This would be a function of the size of the scatterers, since this influences how many can occupy a given volume [12]. The second is the biological variability of the underlying process, that is, the degree to which the process itself varies from one location to another. As an example, we would expect normal connective tissue to be relatively uniform, while calcified plaque would vary significantly from one area to another.

We can measure these effects by examining a histogram of the backscattered amplitude from several different locations of calculating the standard deviation of such measurements [13]. One advantage of such measurements is that they are relative, that is, they do not depend on the absolute backscatter measurement.

Second order statistics. In addition to the statistics

of each sample taken by itself, we can examine the relationship between adjacent values. This can be done by calculating the autocorrelation function, which yields the degree to which samples at various offsets from each other are correlated in value. These values are strongly influenced by the characteristics of the imaging system itself, but also contain some information relating to the second order statistics of the tissue itself. A serious question is to what extent these survive the transformation through the imaging system. This depends primarily on the scale of the tissue variations with respect to the wavelength. Variations much smaller than a wavelength are averaged, and our second order statistics are dominated by the characteristics of the imaging system, primarily the transducer [14].

An alternative method for analyzing such statistics is through arbitrary algorithms such as run length, or texture measures [15]. In general, however, second order statistics are to be preferred, since they can be related directly to the structure of the tissue and transfer function of the imaging system.

Special aspects of intra-arterial tissue characterization

Intra-arterial imaging has several special characteristics when compared with other forms of ultrasound imaging used in cardiology. In almost all cases, the effect of these is to improve the opportunities for ultrasonic tissue characterization.

Probably the single most important factor is that the path from the transducer to the tissue is filled with a relatively uniform fluid, that is blood. This has several fortunate side effects. The primary effect is that there is little attenuation, which allows us to use a high frequency. Another result is that the relatively low attenuation also makes our measurements of backscattered power, for example, less variable due to intervening structures.

High frequency

Since we are able to use higher frequencies, we are able to use shorter pulses, and obtain higher resolution (see section 'Resolution-frequency relationship'). The contribution of structures smaller than the wavelength is also extended towards ever-smaller structures. This is very important, since many of the structures in the cardiovascular system have a mean structural size which is less that the resolution limits for trans-thoracic ultrasound, but amenable to the higher frequencies used in intra-arterial imaging [16].

Types of tissue

An important issue when considering what types of tissue that can be differentiated by ultrasonic tissue characterization is the definition of the fundamental types of interest. Normal muscular wall has several identifiable layers, which can contribute to distinct echoes [17]. We are most interested, however, in pathological tissues comprising plaque. As a first order approximation, we can divide these into normal, fibrous, fibro-fatty, fatty, and calcified [18]. Fibrous tissue is characterized by fibroplasia of the intima, with deposition of collagen, while fatty plaque contains primarily lipid laden cells and cholesterol crystals. Fibrofatty plaque is, logically, a combination of fibrous and fatty plaque, while calcified plaque contains deposits of calcium.

Each of these types of tissue has specific characteristics which could affect the characteristics of the backscattered ultrasound signal. In calcified plaque, the deposits of calcium have a very high reflectivity due to a very large difference in acoustic properties, and the size is relatively large. Fibrous plaque has much finer detail, while fibrofatty plaque contains non-uniformities due to the combination of the two type of tissue. Fatty tissue contains the relatively large structures of fat deposits and cholesterol crystals.

The structures in normal arterial wall are oriented circumferentially, and therefore the reflections from this tissue are anisotropic. As expected, the power of the backscattered signal is greatest when we are perpendicular to the wall, especially for calcified or normal wall, while fibrous plaque shows no significant variability. The magnitude of this variability is about a factor of 10 in power [19]. This will make a difference in the absolute values measured, and must therefore be taken into account.

Transducer design

A significant problem in intra-arterial imaging is the proximity of the structures being imaged. This is because the acoustic field of the transducer is very complex close to its surface, leading to unclear imaging and difficulties in analysis of the signals. The area that this difficulty applies to is called the near field, and its dimensions are not clearly defined. What is clear however, is that a distance within the radius of the transducer face is definitely within the near field.

In building catheters for intra-arterial imaging, we can choose to place the actual transducers on or near the outer surface of the catheter, or place the transducers within the catheter, in some cases using a mirror to further increase this distance. If the transducers are on the surface of the catheter, and we are interested in imaging areas of stenosis, it is inevitable that we will be attempting to image within the near field, with the resulting distortion. Systems which contain a built in offset, via reflecting surfaces, for example, have an advantage in this regard.

Preliminary studies on ultrasonic backscatter from arteries

Although most studies have been done on liver, brain, myocardium, and kidney, there are some studies performed on the backscatter from arterial wall. Most of these are based on lower frequencies than are used in intra-arterial imaging, but provide some valuable indications of potentially productive directions for research.

Absolute backscatter

The easiest parameter to measure in vitro is the total absolute backscatter. A number of studies have shown that the scattering coefficient from normal arterial wall is the smallest, while the backscatter increases from fatty, fibrous, and calcified lesions, in order of increasing intensity [20, 21]. At higher frequencies, the backscattering coefficient from fibrous and calcified tissue can be similar, and therefore difficult to distinguish [22].

Analysis of the detected envelope of the RF signal, using an intraluminal imaging device operating at 20 MHz results in a trend similar to backscattered power measurements at lower frequencies (Fig. 3).

Frequency dependency of backscatter

As noted above, the backscattering coefficient from fibrous tissue and from calcified tissue are very similar. A promising method for distinguishing these two conditions is by analyzing the frequency dependence of the backscatter. The technique is to average the normalized spectra several different sites, and find the slope of the relationship between the frequency and logarithm of backscattered power. This is facilitated by the fact that most imaging transducers have a wide bandwidth, in order to improve radial resolution. A study by Landini [22] of the frequency dependency of backscatter from normal and diseased aortic wall between 4 and 15 MHz showed that only fibrous tissue had an exponent of the frequency dependency of greater than 2.0 (3.3). This is especially encouraging, since this may allow clear distinction between calcified and fibrous lesions. The probable reason for this exponent being less than 4.0, which we would expect with Rayleigh scattering, is the influence of other frequency dependent effects, such as frequency dependent attenuation, and multiple scattering, for example.

182

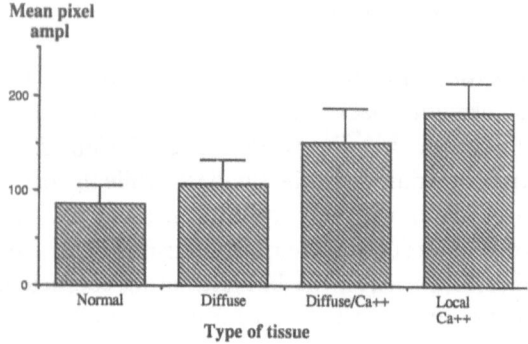

Fig. 3. Comparison of pixel values of detected envelope of backscattered signal in normal artery segments (n = 8), diffusely diseased segments without (n = 7) and with (n = 9) calcium, and localized calcification (n = 10). One hundred pixels were included in each area. The bars are the standard deviation of the pixel values, over all the pixels of a given type. (adapted from Linker [23]).

Frequency dependency of attenuation

The attenuation of various types of arterial wall varies over a wide range, as demonstrated in the study by Picano [18]. The attenuation in calcified tissue is over six times as high as from normal tissue, and the various types of tissue, other than normal and fibrous, do not have values that overlap. The frequency dependence of the attenuation varies even more dramatically, with fatty tissue yielding a slope over 12 times as high as fibrous tissue. In this case, only fatty and calcified tissue were not significantly different.

There are considerable practical problems, however, in measuring attenuation in vivo. In order to make such measurements, we normally must place the receiving transducer on the distal side of the tissue. If we attempt to measure attenuation based on only the backscattered signal, we must make some assumptions about the backscattering coefficient and frequency dependency of backscatter in the tissues distal to the tissue we wish to analyse. It may be possible to use estimation algorithms to reduce the uncertainty of the results [9], but it remains to be seen whether the results are reliable in practice.

First order statistics

Picano [12] studied the backscattered power from normal and diseased aortic wall over a region about 4×4 mm in size, using a 10 MHz transducer. As one would expect, the variance of the backscattered power from region to region varies more in diseased areas than in normal arterial wall. The additional evaluation of skewness and kurtosis allowed distinction of normal from fatty wall.

Linker [23] studied the variance of pixel values in regions of normal and diseased vessel wall, using a 20 MHz intra-arterial imaging system. These results (also shown in Fig. 3) demonstrated an increase in the variance when there was localized or diffuse calcification present.

Acoustic microscopy

As noted in section 'Pulse length and frequency', it is interfaces between tissues of differing acoustic properties which cause the backscattered ultrasound signal. In order to study the structure and distribution of these interfaces, we should use an acoustic microscope [24].

Fig. 4 shows an example of an acoustic micrograph taken from a human muscular artery (iliac), with a fibrous plaque. We can clearly see the relatively homogeneous fibrous tissue, the similar muscular layer, and the very different appearance of the internal and external elastic laminae. This supports the concept that these are the sources of the three layer appearance on intraluminal ultrasound images. Analysis of the spatial distribution of acoustic properties should provide guidelines for future tissue characterization [16].

Elastic properties

Another method of characterizing arterial tissue is not dependent on its ultrasonic scattering properties, but rather on the functional properties. The stiffness of the arterial wall varies as a function of the location in the circulatory system, and disease in the wall. Measures of wall stiffness may related

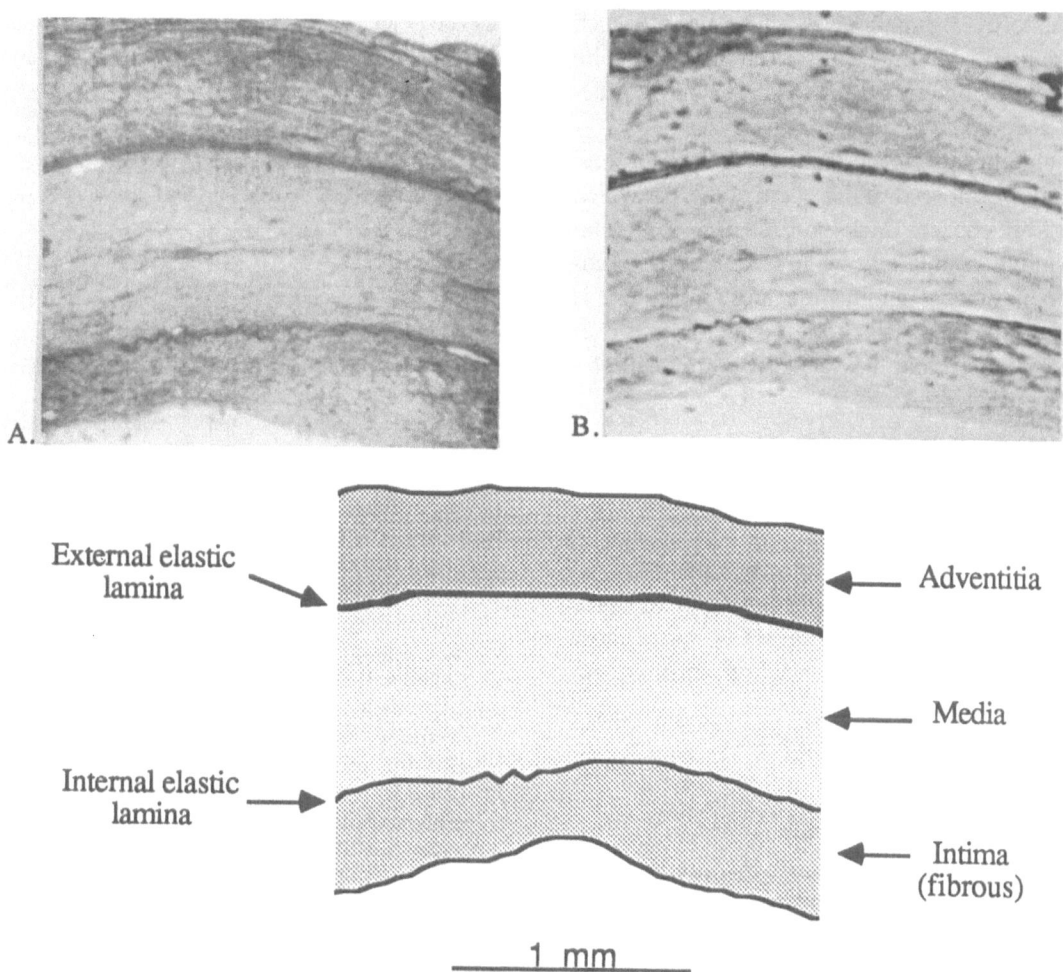

Fig. 4. Reflection light micrograph (A), acoustic micrograph (B), and diagram (C) of a segment of diseased human artery. All are to roughly the same degree of magnification. The acoustic micrograph is taken with a 90 MHz scanning reflection acoustic microscope.

to the mechanism of dilation with balloon angioplasty [25], and differences in wall stiffness in regions of stenosis could alter the response to this and other treatment modalities.

By measuring blood pressure simultaneously with cross sectional imaging, it is possible to calculate wall stress and relate this to the cross sectional dimensions. The slope of this relationship is the wall stiffness [26]. The value obtained must be related to the absolute pressure, since the arterial wall does not obey Hooke's Law, that is, it does not have a linear relationship of stress to strain, but rather increases its stiffness with increasing stress.

Future plans

Clearly, there is much interesting work to be done. Most of the studies cited used frequencies appropriate to non-invasive or intra-operative imaging. It will be necessary to extend these studies to the much higher frequencies used for intra-arterial imaging, at the very least.

The methods described in the preceding sections require alterations in the signal chain, when compared to standard imaging. For operations on the pixel values it is necessary to digitize the video signal, and for more advanced analyses, it is necessary to collect the actual backscattered signal, before detection of the envelope. At present, additional external equipment is necessary for such measurements, but the necessary circuitry could be built into the imaging system to make it more practical in use.

Implementation of the analysis methods in real time may be more difficult, depending on which methods are chosen. Backscattered power is a relatively simple calculation, while frequency dependent attenuation is significantly more complex. It remains to be seen which of the methods are of greatest interest, and how clever we are to implement fast algorithms.

Conclusions

Intra-arterial ultrasound imaging has several unique features which affect the potential for tissue characterization. Most of these make it more likely that practical tissue characterization, in one form or another, will be possible.

References

1. Fraker Jr. TD, Nelson D, Arthur J, Wilkerson RD. Altered acoustic reflectance on two-dimensional echocardiography as an early predictor of myocardial infarct size. Am J Cardiol 1984; 53: 1699–1702.

2. Shaw TRD, Logan-Sinclair RB, Surin C, McAnulty RJ, Heard B, Laurent GJ, Gibson DG. Relation between regional echo intensity and myocardial connective tissue in chronic left ventricular disease Br Heart J 1984; 51: 46–53.

3. Cohen RD, Mottley JG, Miller JG, Kurnik PB, Sobel BE. Detection of ischemic myocardium in vivo through the chest wall by quantitative ultrasonic tissue characterization. Am J Cardiol 1982; 50: 838–43.

4. Yock PG, Johnsen EL, Linker DT. Intravascular ultrasound: Development and clinical potential. Am J Card Imaging 1988; 2(3): 185–93.

5. Roelandt JR, Serruys PW, Bom N, Gussenhoven EJ, van Egmond FC, Lancée CT, ten Hoff H, van Alphen WJ. Intravascular real-time high resolution two-dimensional echocardiography. J Am Coll Card 1989; 13(2): 4A (abstract).

6. Nicholas D. Evaluation of backscattering coefficients for excised human tissues: Results, interpretation and associated measurements. Ultrasound Med Biol 1982; 8(1): 17–28.

7. Rayleigh JWS. The Theory of Sound. Dover Publishers, New York 1896.

8. Parker KJ, Wagg RC. Measurements of ultrasonic attenuation within regions selected from B-scan images. IEEE Trans Biomed Eng BME 1983; 30(8): 431–37.

9 Jang HS, Lee MH, Park SB. Ultrasound attenuation estimation using the LMSE filters and the median filter. Ultrasound in Med & Biol 1988; 14(1): 51–8.

10. Temkin S. Elements of acoustics. John Wiley & Sons, New York 1981.

11. Waag RC, Nilsson JO. Characterization of volume scattering power spectra in isotropic media from power spectra of scattering by planes. J Acoust Soc Am 1982; 74(5): 1555–71.

12. Angelsen BAJ. A theoretical study of the scattering of ultrasound from blood. IEEE Trans Biomed Eng BME 1980; 30(2): 61–7.

13. Picano E, Landini L, Lattanzi F, Mazzarisi A, Sarnelli R, Distante A, Benassi A, L'Abbate A. The use of frequency histograms of ultrasonic backscatter amplitudes for detection of atherosclerosis in vitro. Circ 1986; 74(5): 1093–8.

14. Linker DT, Hansen AS, Tveito Å, Wood J, Torp H, Angelsen BAJ. A two-dimensional simulation of ultrasonic speckle based on acoustic micrographs of human myocardium. In Computers in Cardiology, IEEE Computer Society, Long Beach 1987; 57–61.

15. Collins SM, Skorton DJ, Prasad NV, Olshansky B, Bean JA. Quantitative echocardiographic image texture. Normal contraction related variability. IEEE Trans Med Image 1985; MI-4(4): 185–92.

16. Linker DT, Angelsen BAJ, Popp RL. Acoustic microscopy of normal and myopathic human myocardium: Implications for ultrasonic tissue characterization. J Am Coll Card 1987; 9(2, suppl. A): 211A (abstract).

17. Gussenhoven EJ, Essed CE, Lancée CT, Mastik F, Frietman P, van Egmond FC, Reiber J, Bosch H, van Urk H, Roelandt J, Bom N. Arterial wall characteristics determined by intravascular ultrasound imaging: and in vitro study. J Am Coll Cardiol (in press) 1989.

18. Picano E, Landini L, Distante A, Benassi A, Sarnelli R, L'Abbate A. Fibrosis, lipids, and calcium in human atherosclerotic plaque: In vitro differentiation from normal aortic walls by ultrasonic attenuation. Circ Res 1985; 56: 556–62.

19. Picano E, Landini L, Distante A, Salvadori M, Lattanzi F, Masini M, L'Abbate A. Angle dependence of ultrasonic backscatter in arterial tissues: A study in vitro. Circ 1985; 72(3): 572–6.

20. Picano E, Landini L, Distante A, Sarnelli R, Benassi A, L'Abbate A. Different degrees of atherosclerosis detected by backscattered ultrasound: An in vitro study on fixed human aortic walls. J Clin Ultrasound 1983; 11: 375–9.

21. Barzilai B, Saffitz J, Miller J, Sobel B. Quantitative ultrasonic characterization of the nature of atherosclerotic plaques in human aorta. Circ Res 1987; 60: 459–63.

22. Landini L, Sarnelli R, Picano E, Salvadori M. Evaluation of frequency dependence of backscatter coefficient in normal and atherosclerotic aortic walls. Ultrasound Med & Biol 1986; 12(5): 397–401.

23. Linker DT, Yock PG, Thapliyal HV, Arenson JW, Johansen E, Grønningsæther A, Lønstad HK, Angelsen BAJ. In vitro analysis of backscattered amplitude from normal and diseased arteries using a new intraluminal ultrasonic catheter. J Am Coll Card 1988; 11(2, suppl. A), 4A (abstract).

24. Kolosov OV, Levin VM, Mayev RG, Senjushkina TA. The use of acoustic microscopy for biological tissue characterization. Ultrasound in Med & Biol 1987; 13(8): 477–83.

25. Monsen C, Ambrose JA, Borrico S, Cohen M, Sherman W, Gorlin R, Fuster V. Patterns of dilation during coronary angioplasty. J Am Coll Cardiol 1989; 13(2): 58A (abstract).

26. Linker DT, Johansen E, Slørdal S, Yock PG, Grønningsæter Å, Peine H, Angelsen BAJ. In vivo measurement of segmental arterial wall stiffness in pigs using a real-time ultrasonic sector imaging catheter. J Am Coll Card 1989; 13(2, suppl. A): 218 A (abstract).

International Journal of Cardiac Imaging 4: 187–193, 1989.
© 1989 *Kluwer Academic Publishers*.

Clinical percutaneous imaging of coronary anatomy using an over-the-wire ultrasound catheter system

J. McB. Hodgson, S.P. Graham, A.D. Savakus, S.G. Dame, D.N. Stephens, P.S. Dhillon, D. Brands,
H. Sheehan & M.J. Eberle
*Division of Cardiology, McGuire VAMC and Medical College of Virginia, 1201 Broad Rock Boulevard,
Richmond, VA 23249, USA*

Abstract

This manuscript describes initial applications of a unique new intravascular ultrasound imaging catheter. This 5.5F catheter uses an over-the-wire design and incorporates a phased array transducer at its tip. There are no moving parts. A 360° image is produced perpendicular to the catheter axis using a 20 MHz center frequency. A dedicated minicomputer is used for initial image processing, as well as enhancement and analysis. Initial studies using phantoms demonstrated excellent accuracy for linear dimensions (r = 0.99, range 3.0 to 7.6 mm, image = 1.0 phantom + 0.1). Serial imaging of the same arterial segment in vitro showed good reproducibility (coefficients of variance 2.5–5.2%). Likewise, intra- and inter-observer variability in image analysis was minimal (r = 0.92–0.99). Initial in vivo studies were performed in dogs. The catheter was easily passed over a wire into mesenteric, cerebral and coronary vessels without evidence of significant vessel trauma. Subsequently, 20 patients had percutaneous coronary imaging performed during cardiac catheterization. Cardiac motion was rarely a problem and acceptable images were obtained in all but two patients. Areas of calcification, mild stenoses, branching vessels and graft atherosclerosis could be identified. We conclude that intracoronary ultrasound imaging will be useful for assessing vascular pathology, for studying both rapid change in vessel size as well as chronic progression or regression of atherosclerosis, and for assisting with new therapeutic interventions.

Introduction

Until recently, contrast angiography has been the gold standard for assessing coronary anatomy and disease processes which affect the coronaries. Despite advances in digital processing [1, 2], angiography has been unable to yield reliable information about arterial wall morphology [3, 4]. Angioscopy has allowed detailed study of the endothelial surface of the coronaries in conscious patients [5, 6]. Such study has enhanced our understanding of complex atherosclerotic processes as well as the injury produced by therapeutic interventions. Angioscopy, however, is unable to yield information about vessel wall thickness and is poorly suited for dimensional measurements. Intravascular ultra-sound is a new technology which provices an alternative method of studying arterial structure. Initial studies were performed using intra-operative epicardial probes [7, 8]. More recently, catheter mounted transducers have allowed real time percutaneous transluminal imaging in conscious patients [9–12]. We, and others, have reported good correlation between ultrasound images and histologic vessel sections [13–15], the potential for angioplasty and atherectomy guidance [16–18], the ability to visualize thrombus [19] and intimal flaps [20] and the capacity to study beat-to-beat changes in arterial cross-sectional area [21]. These capabilities make intravascular ultrasound an attractive adjunct to current diagnostic and therapeutic modalities in addition to providing new capabilities suited for both acute and chronic study of the vasculature. This manuscript describes initial validation and preliminary percutaneous coronary imaging studies in patients using an over-the-wire, phased array ultrasound catheter.

Methods

Technical details of the catheter

The ultrasound catheter incorporates a polyethylene shaft and a phased array transducer tip (Endosonics Cathscanner Model 301, Rancho Cordova, CA). The greatest width is 5.5 F (1.83 mm) at the tip with reduction to a 4.5 F shaft. A central lumen accomodates a 0.014″ guidewire. The catheter fits easily through a 9 F large lumen guide (ID = 0.088″, Interventional Medical, Danvers, Mass). The transducer operates at a center frequency of 20 MHz. The multi-element array yields an image perpendicular to the axis of the catheter as depicted in Fig. 1.

Initial processing is done at the transducer tip using integrated circuits with subsequent processing in a dedicated minicomputer. The field of view is operator adjustable from 8 to 16 mm in diameter and images may be acquired up to 10 frames/second. Digital processing allows the image to be optimally focused at each point along the radial axis. Patient interface is made through a pin connector and battery powered, isolated pre-processing unit which may be positioned in the sterile field. Fiberoptic connections between the patient unit and computer ensure low interference and isolation integrity. A dedicated interface is provided for physician control of image depth, scan rates, grey levels, enhancement features and analysis options. Images are recorded on video tape for immediate review. A radio-opaque distal tip marker allows for precise localization during fluoroscopy.

In vitro analysis – Phantoms

A phantom of low density polyethylene with previously drilled holes of known diameters ranging

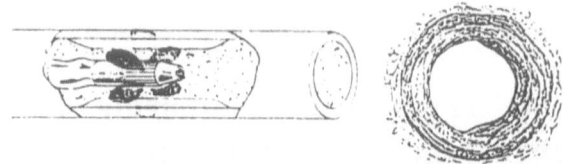

Fig. 1. Artist's sketch showing the ultrashound catheter in a vessel (left). The transducer elements are arranged circumferentially about the tip. The ultrasound beam is projected perpendicular to the long axis of the catheter and produces a cross-sectional image as depicted to the right.

from 3 to 7.5 mm was imaged in a saline bath. The catheter was positioned by hand to obtain a coaxial image using real time scan rates.

In vitro analysis – Vascular tissue

Dimensional comparisons of ultrasound and histologic sections have been reported previously [13]. We performed additional studies to determine the influence of blood as an imaging medium. Excised, fixed human vessels were imaged in normal saline and again in citrated blood (hematocrit 35%). Additionally, the reproducibility of repeated imaging was investigated. For analysis of scan reproducibility, the same vascular sample was imaged using five separate catheter placements (hand positioning). For histologic analysis, vessel segments were sectioned and processed using standard decalcification, paraffin embedding and staining techniques. Photographs of the histologic sections were obtained using 35 mm black and white film.

Image analysis

Histologic photographic images and corresponding ultrasound images were digitized using an image processing computer (ADAC DPS 4100C, Milpitas, CA) and analyzed using standard algorithms for lumen diameter, lumen cross-sectional area, total vessel area, wall thickness and wall area. For calibration, ultrasound images were scaled using the phantom block. Histologic samples were calibrated using a ruler photographed with each sample.

To assess inter-observer variability, two observers analyzed the same images. To assess intra-observer variability, one observer analyzed the same images on two occasions separated by at least 2 days.

In vivo analysis

To assess catheter handling characteristics and safety with regard to vessel trauma, initial studies were performed in animals. Mongrel dogs (20–34 kg) of either sex (n = 8) were anesthetized using sodium thiamyal (35 mg/kg) and ventilated with oxygen enriched room air. Aortic pressure and electrocardiogram were monitored continuously. A 9 F sheath was percutaneously placed in the right femoral artery. A 9 F guiding catheter was positioned at the orifice of the vessel to be imaged. An 0.014″ angioplasty guidewire was then advanced into the vessel and the imaging catheter advanced over the wire to the desired scanning location. A combination of wire, guide and catheter manipulation was used to align the catheter coaxial in the vessel for optimal imaging. Following imaging, the animal was sacrificed and arterial segments were perfusion fixed at 100 mmHg using 2% glutaraldehyde. After standard paraffin embedding, sections were taken longitudinally through the vessel and stained with hematoxylin and eosin. Sections were then assessed for vessel wall trauma. This protocol was approved by the Animal Care and Use Committee, Medical College of Virginia and the McGuire VAMC Research and Development Committee.

Patient studies

Twenty patients underwent percutaneous intracoronary ultrasound imaging. These patients gave written informed consent and were undergoing cardiac catheterization for clinical indications. Patients with significantly stenotic (> 50%) or diffusely diseased coronaries were excluded. Imaging was performed using 9 F guiding catheters and 0.014″ floppy guidewires. The imaging catheter was advanced over the wire into the right, left anterior descending and circumflex coronaries and aortocoronary bypass grafts. This protocol was approved by the Human Studies Committee of Virginia Commonwealth University and the McGuire VAMC Research and Development Committee.

Statistics

Correlations between histologic and ultrasound images were calculated using linear regression. Inter- and intra-observer variability were assessed by linear regression. Reproducibility was calculated as coefficients of variance. Values of $p < 0.05$ were considered significant. Data are expressed as mean ± standard error of the mean.

Results

In vitro – Phantoms

The accuracy of ultrasound image dimensions over the range of 3.0 mm to 7.5 mm was excellent (Fig. 2). Repeated determinations (n = 7) at each phantom diameter were consistent. Coefficients of variance ranged from 7% (at 3 mm) to 2% (at 7.5 mm).

In vitro: Blood-saline comparison

Comparison of blood and saline as imaging media showed close correlation for all dimensional data (Table 1). There was some decrease in signal when imaging was performed in blood as compared to saline, however, this did not interfere with image analysis.

Reproducibility of ultrasound imaging

Serial ultrasound images of the same arterial segment (5 independent probe placements) demonstrated excellent reproducibility of image and dimensional data (Table 2).

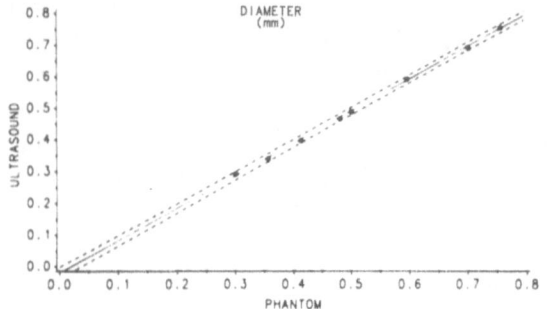

Fig. 2. Correlation between known phantom block diameters and ultrasound image determined diameters. (r = 0.99, image = 1.0 phantom + 0.1).

Reproducibility of image analysis

The correlations for all operator derived dimensions were excellent for both intra- and inter-observer determinations (Table 3).

Table 1. Comparison of imaging in blood and saline

Parameters	Vessels imaged	Correlation coefficient (r)	Mean value
Lumen area (mm^2)	12	0.98	38.5 ± 8.8
Maximal lumen diamater (mm)	12	0.95	8.5 ± 0.5
Wall area (mm^2)	12	0.91	67.3 ± 6.0
Maximal wall thickness (mm)	12	0.96	2.5 ± 0.1

In vivo performance and safety

The ultrasound catheter was easily passed over an 0.014″ angioplasty guide wire into the cerebral, mesenteric and pelvic vessels. Flexibility was excellent and fluoroscopic visualization of the distal tip marker was adequate. By manipulation of the catheter, guide wire and guide catheter, coaxial images could be obtained.

Table 2. Scan reproducibility

Parameter	# Scans per vessel	# Vessels imaged	Average coefficient of variance	Range
Lumen area	5	9	3.3 ± 1.2%	(1.1–5.1)
Minimal lumen diameter	5	9	2.5 ± 1.3%	(0.8–4.1)
Maximal lumen diameter	5	9	2.6 ± 0.7%	(1.9–3.9)
Wall area	5	8	4.0 ± 2.4%	(0.8–7.4)
Maximal wall thickness	5	7	5.2 ± 1.7%	(2.5–7.1)

Table 3. Variability of ultrasound image analysis

	Correlation between observations			
	Lumen area	Lumen diameter maximum	Wall area	Wall thickness maximum
Intra-observer				
r	0.98	0.96	0.99	0.94
n	18	19	22	13
Inter-observer				
r	0.99	0.99	0.98	0.92
n	47	42	30	30

There were no complications related to catheter use. Perfusion fixed histologic sections from arteries imaged by the catheter showed mild endothelial denudation (< 25% of examined area) with occasional subintimal hemorrhage.

Patient studies

Adequate images were obtained in all but two patients (n = 20). There were no complications. In general, images appeared to have a single wall layer of approximately 1.0–2.0 mm in thickness (Fig. 3).

In some patients, a three layered appearance suggestive of diffuse fibrous plaque was observed even when the associated angiogram appeared normal (Fig. 4). Branch points could be easily identified (Fig. 5). Fig. 6 displays a normal appearing mid left anterior descending segment (left) adjacent to an area of mild stenosis (right). Mild stenoses were characterized by decreased lumen area and thick walls. Diffuse graft atherosclerosis appeared as bright echo reflections and thickened walls (Fig. 7).

Discussion

The major finding of these studies is that percutaneous intracoronary ultrasound imaging may be accomplished safely in patients using an over-the-wire phased array catheter. Additionally, we have demonstrated accuracy and reproducibility of dimensional image data and lack of significant catheter induced vascular trauma in animals.

Patient studies confirmed the ease of wire tracking and flexibility observed in the animal studies. Imaging allowed identification of wall thickness, lumen area, branch points, calcification and mild stenoses. Due to the real time imaging capabilities, ultrasound imaging will also allow rapid changes in arterial vasomotor tone to be followed.

Potential limitations of this catheter include a somewhat large profile (5.5 F) making passage into smaller coronary branches (< 2 mm) or through significant stenoses impossible. Work is currently underway to provide both a smaller version for

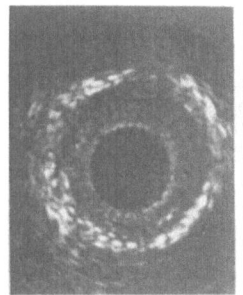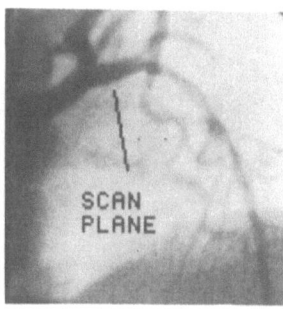

Fig. 3. Intraluminal ultrasound image obtained in the left anterior descending artery (left). The internal and adventitial borders are seen. The catheter appears as a black circle in the center of the vessel. The corresponding angiogram displaying the image scan plane is shown to the right.

intracoronary work as well as a larger version for peripheral vascular applications. It was important to maintain the catheter coaxial in the vessel to obtain the highest quality image. This requirement is not unique to the phased array design. Angulation of more than 10–15° from the centerline of the vessel results in serious image degradation for both phased array and mechanical [9] imaging catheters. Work is underway to provide some steering capability for the catheter used in this study. Such capabilities will greatly improve the ability to image at any desired location in the vessel. The phased array

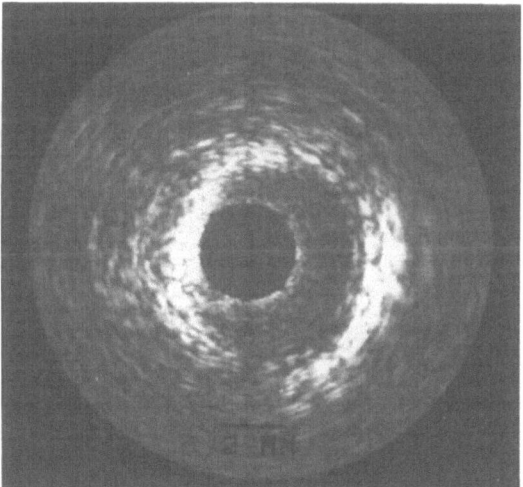

Fig. 4. A three layered appearance is evident in this left anterior descending coronary. Prior histologic studies have shown this pattern to correspond to early fibrous atherosclerotic lesions [13].

192

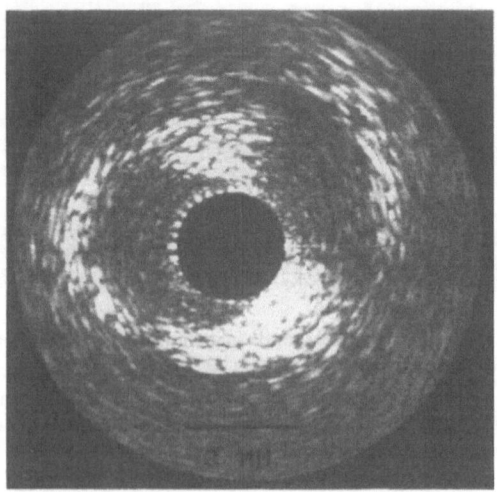

Fig. 5. This image of a left main coronary demonstrates the origin of the circumflex artery in the 2 : 00 position.

design is associated with a lower signal to noise ratio than single transducer mechanical catheters. Again, the prototype catheters used in this study are undergoing continual design modifications which promise to significantly enhance current signal to noise ratios.

A potential advantage of the phased array design is greater control over image processing and focus-ing. The major advantages of the phased array design, however, are the ability to easily accomodate a guide wire lumen and the small distal tip with associated flexible shaft. This design allows for easy incorporation of the transducer tip into other interventional devices such as balloon angioplasty catheters, atherectomy catheters, or lasers. The imaging tip can also be easily combined with pressure and/or velocity sensors.

We conclude, based on these preliminary studies, that percutaneous intravascular ultrasound imaging will contribute significantly to the modalities currently available for the study of vascular pathology. Likewise, this technology is well suited for the assessment of acute or chronic changes in arterial dimensions, wall thickness or lumen area. Finally, ultrasound imaging may prove useful for the assessment of therapeutic interventions such as angiography, atherectomy or laser ablation.

References

1. Mancini G, Simon G, McGillem MJ, LeFree M, Friedman H, Vogel R. Automated quantitative coronary arteriography: morphologic and physiologic validation in vivo of a rapid digital angiographic method. Circulation 1987; 75: 452–60.

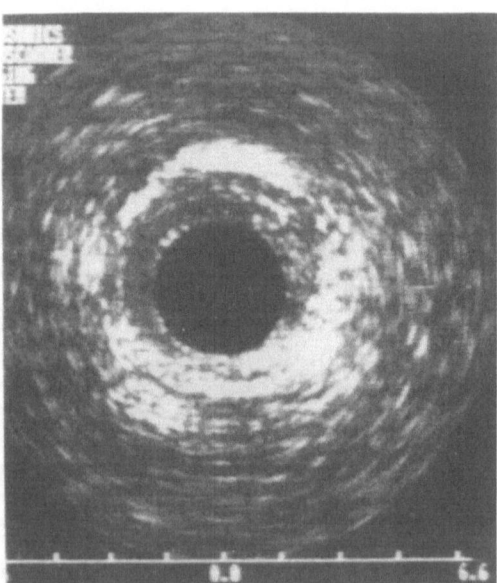

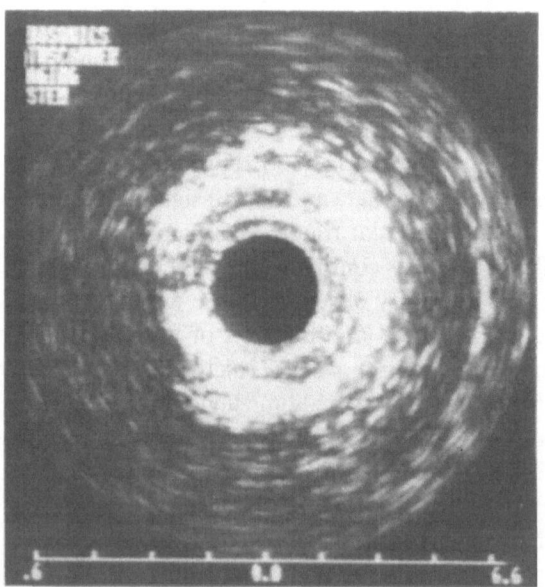

Fig. 6. These images demonstrate a more normal segment (left) and a stenotic segment (right).

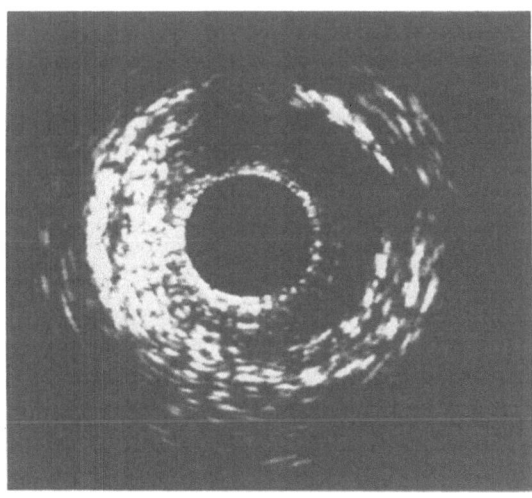

Fig. 7. Thickened walls and multiple reflectors are seen in this image of a diseased aorto-coronary bypass graft.

mond F, Lancee C, ten Hoff H, van Alphen W. Intravascular real-time, high resolution two-dimensional echocardiography. (Abst) J Am Coll Cardiol 1989; 13: 4A.

10. Yock P, Linker D, Saether O, Thapliyal H, Arenson J, White N, Ports T, Angelsen B. Intravascular two-dimensional catheter ultrasound: initial clinical studies. (Abst) Circulation 1988; 78(II): II-21.

11. Pandian N, Kreis A, Desnoyers M, Isner J, Salem D, Sacharoff A, Boleza E, Wilson R, Caro R. In vivo ultrasound angioscopy in humans and animals: intraluminal imaging of blood vessels using a new catheter-based high resolution ultrasound probe. (Abst) Circulation 1988;78(II): II-22.

12. Hodgson J, Graham S, Savakus A. Percutaneous intravascular ultrasound imaging in humans: initial peripheral and coronary studies. (Abst) J Am Soc Echo 1989 (in press).

13. Hodgson J, Eberle M, Savakus A. Validation of a new real-time percutaneous intrasound intravascular ultrasound imaging catheter. (Abst) Circulation 1988; 78(II): II-21.

14. Pandian NG, Kreis A, Brockway B, Isner JM, Sacharoff A, Boleza E, Caro R, Muller D. Ultrasound angioscopy: real-time, two-dimensional, intraluminal ultrasound imaging of blood vessels. Am J Cardiol 1988; 62: 493–4.

15. Bartorelli A, Potkin B, Almagor Y, Gessert J, Roberts W, Leon M. Intravascular ultrasound imaging of atherosclerotic coronary arteries: an in vitro validation study. (Abst) J Am Cardiol 1989; 13: 4A.

16. Tobis J, Mallery J, Gessert J, Griffith J, Bessen M, Macleay L, Morcos N, Henry W. Intravascular ultrasound visualization before and after balloon angioplasty. (Abst) Circulation 1988; 78(II): II-84.

17. Tobis J, Mallery J, Mahon D, Griffith J, Gessert J, Macleay L, Mcrae M, Bessen M, Henry W. Intravascular ultrasound visualization of atheroma plaque removal by atherectomy. (Abst) J Am Coll Cardiol 1989; 13: 222A.

18. Graham S, Brands D, Savakus A, Hodgson J. Utility of an intravascular ultrasound imaging device for arterial wall definition and atherectomy guidance. (Abst) J Am Coll Cardiol 1989; 13: 222A.

19. Pandian N, Kreis A, Brockway B, Sacharoff A, Boleza E, Caro R. Detection of intravascular thrombus by high frequency intraluminal ultrasound angioscopy: in vitro and in vivo studies. (Abst) J Am Coll Cardiol 1989; 13: 5A.

20. Pandian N, Kreis A, Brockway B, Sacharoff A, Boleza E, Caro R. Intraluminal ultrasound angioscopic detection of arterial dissection and intimal flaps: in vitro and in vivo studies. (Abst) Circulation 1988; 78(II): II-21.

21. Hodgson J, Graham S, Savakus A. Usefulness of Doppler and ultrasound imaging catheters for assessing rapid changes incoronary flow and artery area. (Abst) J Am Soc Echo 1989 (in press).

2. Spears J, Sandor T, Als A, et al. Computerized image analysis for quantitative measurement of vessel diameter from cineangiograms. Circulation 1983; 68: 453–61.

3. Grondin C, Dyrda I, Pasternac A, Campean L, Bourassa M, Lesperance J. Discrepancies between cineangiographic and postmortem findings in patients with coronary artery disease and recent myocardial revascularization. Circulation 1974; 49: 703–8.

4. Arnett E, Isner J, Redwood D, et al. Coronary artery narrowing in coronary heart disease: Comparison of cineangiographic and necropsy findings. Ann Intern Med 1979; 91: 350–6.

5. Sherman C, Litvack F, Grundfest W, et al. Coronary angioscopy in patients with unstable angina pectoris. N Engl J Med 1986; 315: 913–9.

6. Grundfest W, Litvack F, Sherman T, et al. Delineation of peripheral and coronary detail by intraoperative angioscopy. Ann Surg 1985; 202: 394–400.

7. Johnson M, McPherson D, Fleagle S, et al. Videodensitometric analysis of human coronary stenosis: validation in vivo by intraoperative high-frequency epicardial echocardiography. Circulation 1988; 77: 328–36.

8. Sahn D, Copeland J, Temkin L, Wirt D, Mammana R, Glenn W. Anatomic-ultrasound correlations for intraoperative open chest imaging of coronary artery atherosclerotic lesions in human beings. J Am Coll Cardiol, 1984; 3: 1169–77.

9. Roelandt J, Serruys P, Bom N, Gussenhoven J, van Eg-

International Journal of Cardiac Imaging **4**: 195–199, 1989.

Imaging artifacts in mechanically driven ultrasound catheters

H. ten Hoff[1], A. Korbijn[2], Th.H.Smit[2], J.F.F. Klinkhamer[3], N. Bom[1,4]
[1] *Thoraxcentre, Erasmus University Rotterdam,* [2] *University of Technology Delft,* [3] *Produktcentrum TNO and* [4] *Interuniversity Cardiology Institute of the Netherlands, P.O. Box 1738, 3000 DR Rotterdam, the Netherlands*

Abstract

Mechanically driven catheter tip echo systems presently operate with a flexible shaft. Rotation power from a proximally mounted motor is transferred via this shaft to the rotating echo tip element. In practice, the tip does not identically 'follow' the rotation of the motor due to low torsional rigidity of the shaft, which creates artifacts in the displayed cross-sectional image. In order to visualize curved arteries such as the coronary arteries, a compromise is necessary between the required low flexural rigidity and a high torsional rigidity.

In this report the image artifacts of mechanically driven systems are presented that are related to catheter tip motion. The properties of a spiral drive-shaft and a solid drive-shaft have been compared for rotational speed of 1000 and 3000 revolutions per minute (rpm), and for straight as well as strongly curved catheters. By way of example, the periodic angle error varies from 25 degrees top-top in a straight catheter to 80 degrees top-top when the catheter is curved with R = 20 mm, using a spiral drive-shaft at 1000 rpm.

Introduction

The principle of ultrasound (US-) catheter imaging and the medical need for these devices have been discussed in the previous chapters. In these systems echo image quality is important. Not only should the vessel cross-section be displayed with the proper gray-scale, but geometrical distortion in the visualization process should be reliably avoided.

For a proper interpretation of the image, knowledge of artifacts must be available. These artifacts are in part caused by the physics of echo acoustics and are well known in diagnostic ultrasound. They include attenuation, reverberation, shadowing etc. A second class of artifacts may be caused by the physical properties of the catheter such as tip motion or error in display angle in mechanically rotated echo tip systems. This chapter is limited to the latter class of artifacts. The US-imaging system being dealt with here is schematically illustrated in Fig. 1. It contains a flexible drive-shaft for rotational scanning. This principle is used by most of the developers of US-imaging catheters.

The flexible drive-shaft is rotated by a motor at the proximal side of the catheter. The shaft transfers this rotational motion to the US-transducer at the distal catheter-tip. In order to achieve real-time imaging, the velocity of rotation typically ranges from 1000 to 3000 rpm.

Image artifacts related to catheter tip motion

Image artifacts related to catheter tip motion are image distortion and lack of resolution due to angular and radial position uncertainties of the US-transducer in relation to the imaged tissue structures. In particular the angular position error has been studied for two classes of drive-shafts of varying flexibility.

Angular position uncertainty

If a uniform rotation is applied to the proximal side of the drive-shaft, the distal side will exhibit a non-

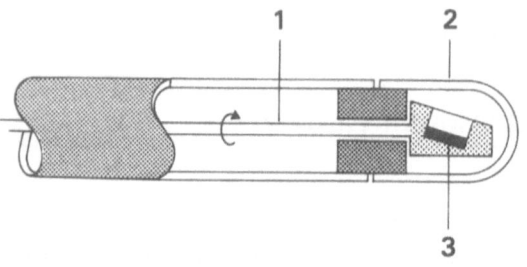

Fig. 1. Principle of mechanically rotated catheter tip echo transducer. Flexible drive-shaft (1), sonolucent dome (2), piezo transducer (3).

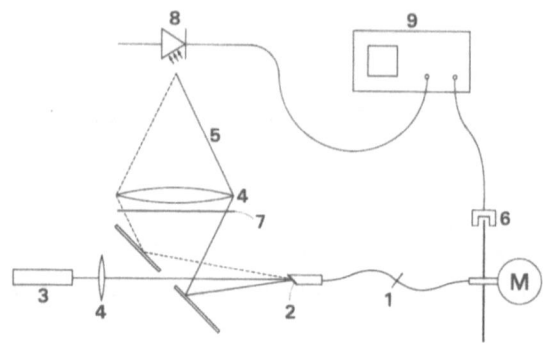

Fig. 2. Set-up for testing drive-shaft angular performance. 1. Flexible drive-shaft in catheter tube; 2. Rotating mirror; 3. Laser; 4. Positive lens; 5. Rotating light beam; 6. Proximal angular encoder; 7. Distal angular encoder; 8. Photo-detector; 9. Angular decoder/data processing.

uniform motion. This is due to unavoidable friction of the drive-shaft in the enclosing catheter tube and in the bearing at the tip, combined with the limited torsional rigidity of the drive-shaft. The demand for a flexible catheter and thus flexible drive-shaft conflicts with the need for maximum torsional rigidity of the shaft. Compromising in this matter will increase the angular uncertainty of the transducer-tip. It is easy to measure the rotation angle at the proximal side of the shaft. It is much more difficult to know the precise angle at the distal tip. Under worst case conditions stick-slip may occur. This means that the transducer comes to a full-stop followed by very fast acceleration. If the angular information from the proximal side of the shaft is used exclusively to create the echo image, image distortion will occur. The angle on the display may not correspond faithfully to the angle of the transducer sound beam and will thus create distorted or blurred images.

Experiments for testing the mechanical performance of certain catheter-drive-shaft combinations under given curved conditions, using the set-up shown in Fig. 2, have shown that the differences between proximal and distal angular position can be substantial. As a result, important loss of image quality must be expected.

The catheter and shaft (1) are curved according to a set of standard and realistic curvatures. These range from straight, via R = 200 mm curvature, up to a curvature of R = 20 mm. Rotational speed can be varied from 1000 to 3000 rpm. At the tip of the shaft, a small mirror (2) is mounted. A laser light source (3) and beam focussing lens (4) are shown to the left in Fig. 2. The light beam is rotated and

projected through a circular code disk (7) having 200 radial lines, onto a second lens (4) which focusses the light beam onto a diode (8). At a given moment the light beam is represented by the drawn line. The dashed line represents the light beam a little later in time, after 180° rotation of mirror (2). A comparison between the proximal encoder signal (6), which also contains 200 pulses per revolution, and the distal encoder signal is performed in processing unit 9.

The angular error has three components, each having its own effect on the image quality. A constant error represents a constant difference in angular position between proximal and distal side. This error only affects the relationship of angular orientation between the image and the actual vessel cross-section. It does not influence image quality as such; the result is a 'misorientation'.

The periodic error represents a non-uniform motion of the distal side with periodic components related to the periodicity of rotation. This error does cause image distortion (see Fig. 3).

One can misjudge the angular extent of a vascular wall process. In sectors of high angular speed, information from a broader angle will be collected than will be displayed on screen. Conversely at low speed the image will be subject to angular expansion. The periodic error will not cause image blurring since in every revolution of the transducer the corresponding image lines will coincide.

Superimposed on these two errors a stochastic

COMPRESSION

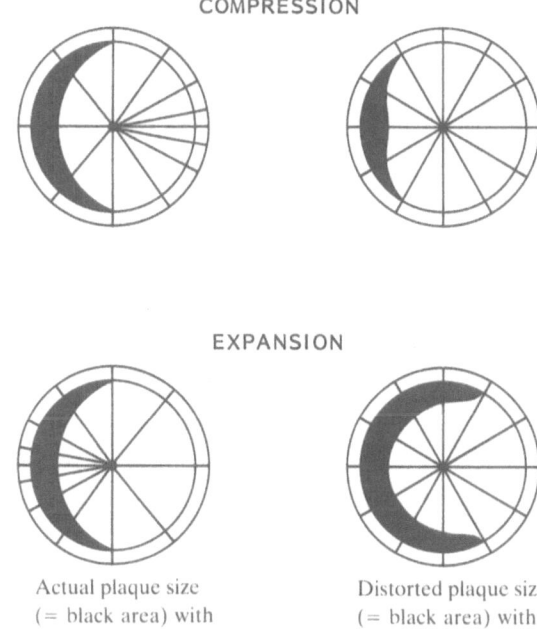

EXPANSION

Actual plaque size
(= black area) with
US-beam directions

Distorted plaque size
(= black area) with
image lines

Fig. 3. Effect of periodic angular error on image quality: angular distortion (compression and expansion).

error may occur. This results in a misalignment of corresponding image lines from succeeding revolutions which creates a blurred image.

We examined two types of flexible drive-shafts: a 100 cm long flexible, spiral drive-shaft with limited torsional rigidity (flexural rigidity = 14 Nmm^2; torsional rigidity = 27 Nmm^2) and a 120 cm long, less flexible, solid tube drive-shaft with high torsional rigidity (flexural rigidity = 466 Nmm^2; torsional rigidity = 368 Nmm^2).

In Fig. 4, the two most serious errors (the periodic and stochastic errors) are shown for three particular cases, using the spiral type drive-shaft. The measurements were performed with the use of the set-up depicted in Fig. 2.

In this figure, the error between the distal and proximal rotation angle is plotted versus the proximal rotation angle. The solid line represents the periodic error variation over a constant angular error 'C'. The 90% probability range is indicated by the dotted lines and represents the stochastic error.

It can be seen from these figures that the motion behaviour of the rotating tip is changed by the

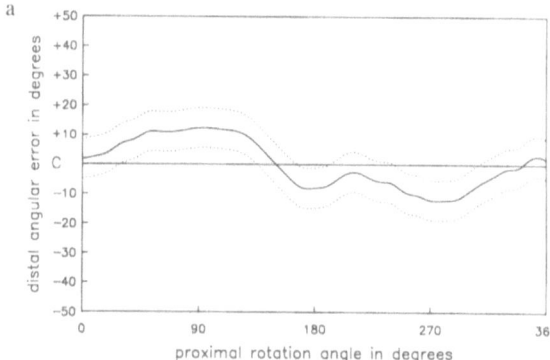

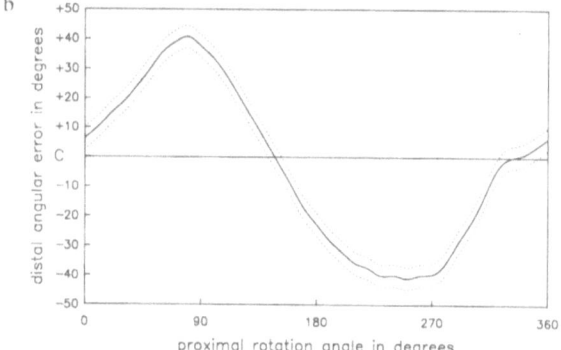

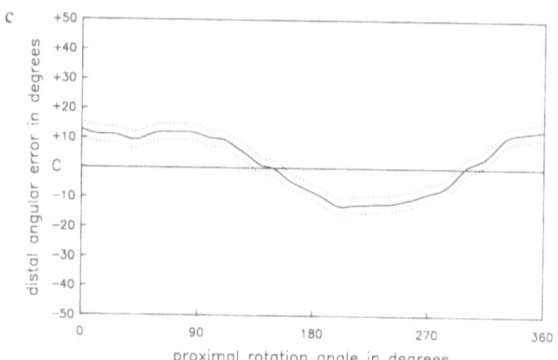

Fig. 4. Angular error over the spiral type drive-shaft. a. A straight catheter at 1000 rpm; b. A 90° curved catheter, with R = 20 mm, at 1000 rpm; c. A 90° curved catheter, with R = 20 mm, at 3000 rpm.
C = level of constant angular error
—— = periodic angular error
..... = stochastic angular error; 90% probability range

application of a severe curve at the distal end of the catheter. The periodic error will increase, probably due to the increasing dynamic friction, the value of which will fluctuate periodically.

The non-periodic stochastic error component decreases, possibly due to decreasing freedom of motion of the drive-shaft caused by the increasing friction at the tip.

Increasing the velocity of rotation improves the mechanical performance of the drive-shaft. This may be caused by decreasing friction and the fact that the occurrence of stick-slip is less probable.

In Fig. 5 the combination of periodic and stochastic angular errors as measured using a solid tube type drive-shaft in the set-up of Fig. 2 is illustrated.

Figs. 4a and 5a show that under straight circumstances the performance of the torsionally rigid solid tube type drive-shaft is much better than that of the flexible spiral shaft. Periodic and stochastic angular errors of the latter are twice the size of the errors of the first. But if the catheter is also used under curved conditions the performance of the solid tube shaft will decline rapidly (see Fig. 5b). Application of curvatures with R < 100 mm is not realistic for the use in blood vessels because of the high bending moments that are needed. Furthermore the use of high speed rotation combined with curvatures of R < 200 mm will lead to the breakdown of the shaft by fatigue.

High speed continuous drive versus stepping motion

The angular position of the transducer changes between the moment of emitting and receiving the ultrasonic signals. Assuming a typical maximum penetration depth of 10 mm the angle between the two transducer positions will be 0.08 degrees per 1000 rpm. The US-beam emitted in one specific direction has some angular dispersion so that the transducer in the new receiving position will be most sensitive to echoes from the less central parts of the emitted beam. This means that information is collected along radial lines slightly curved in the direction of rotation, but presently is displayed on the screen along straight radial lines (see Fig. 6).

At very high rates of rotation (> 10,000 rpm), the angle between emitting and receiving position of the transducer sound beam becomes so large that the transducer only receives echoes reflected

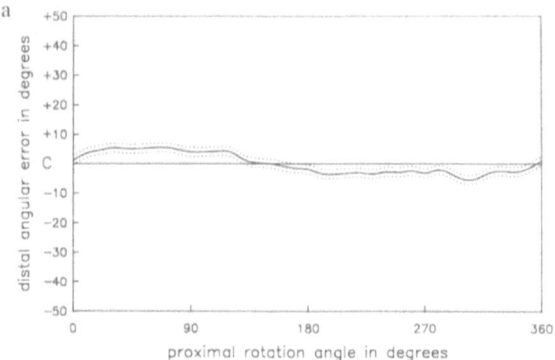

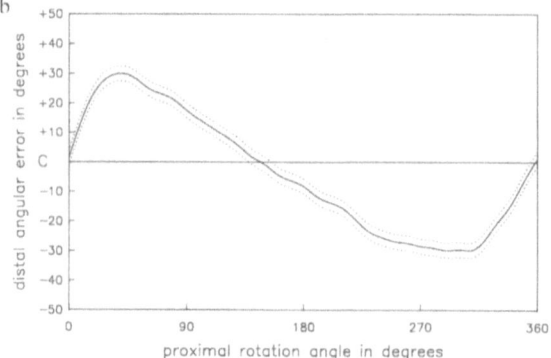

Fig. 5. Angular error over a solid tube type drive-shaft with rotational speed of 1000 rpm. a. A straight catheter; b. A 90° curved catheter with R = 100 mm.

c = level of constant angular error

——— = periodic angular error

..... = stochastic angular error; 90% probability range

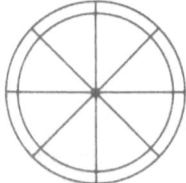
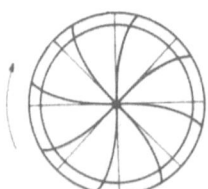

Stepping motion; echo info collected along straight lines.

High speed continuous drive; echo info collected along curved lines.

Fig. 6. Angular image distortion due to continuous high speed rotation of the transducer.

at greater depth, from directions deviating substantially from the acoustic beam axis. This will cause a loss of sensitivity.

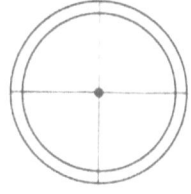 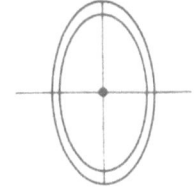

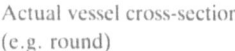

Actual vessel cross-section US-image (ellipsoid)
(e.g. round)

Fig. 7. The effect of periodic lateral catheter-tip motion on the image quality.

Radial position uncertainty

Because of the rotating drive-shaft in the catheter tube lateral movement of the catheter-tip may occur. Again this motion will be a combination of a periodic component related to the periodicity of rotation, and a stochastic one. The first causes image distortion, which easily can escape notice, but can lead to false conclusions about the vessel cross-section (see Fig. 7). The latter diminishes the radial resolution in real-time imaging.

Errors due to vessel wall motion

A second source of radial position errors is given by the vessel wall motion caused by the pulsatile blood flow. One image frame should be created within a small fraction of a heart cycle to overcome this problem. The minimum rate of rotation is approximately 1000 rpm to limit wall motion artifacts to an acceptable level.

The pulsatile wall motion also causes lateral motion of the catheter tip. The image on the display will move accordingly if its center represents the catheter position. Fast computational correction on the display is a possible solution for this behaviour.

Conclusions

In order to interpret the echo images correctly, distortion should be minimized or at least artifacts should be fully understood. The diagnostic catheter may serve various clinical applications, and some of these will demand a highly flexible catheter. It has been shown that this results in a discrepancy between the displayed echo beam and the real echo beam position. As a result image distortion is introduced. We have shown that for a highly flexible drive-shaft this angle error can be many degrees.

The solution to this problem would be the introduction of an angle coding technique at the tip position.

Acknowledgements

Construction of our catheter prototype has been carried out by Produktcentrum TNO and TPD-TNO at Delft, the Netherlands and the Central Research Workshop of the Erasmus University Rotterdam. The investigations are supported by the Netherlands Technology Foundation (STW) and the Dutch Ministry of Economic Affairs.

International Journal of Cardiac Imaging **4**: 201–216, 1989.
© 1989 *Kluwer Academic Publishers.*

Design characteristics for intravascular ultrasonic catheters

Roy W. Martin[1] & Christopher C. Johnson[2]
[1] Department of Anesthesiology/Center for Bioengineering University of Washington, RN-10, Seattle, WA 98195 USA; [2] Division of Cardiology, University of Washington & Veterans Administration Medical Center, RG-22, Seattle, WA 98195 USA

Abstract

Several factors are important in the design of intracoronary ultrasonic imaging catheters. The mechanical considerations are first discussed and equations are developed for calculating the forces affecting catheter passage in a blood vessel. These equations are applied to the problem of Judkins (transfemoral) coronary artery catheterization, using previously described anatomical information and catheter moduli values. The introduction force is calculated for each position along the vessel for both a high and low value of estimated catheter-wall friction (coefficient values of 0.04 and 0.2, respectively). Next, the problem of catheter or transducer rotation is analytically described. The advantages of spiral drive cables with high torsional rigidity and low bending stiffness are numerically shown. Finally, several methods and considerations are given for electrical connection to the transducer. These results and equations should facilitate the design of intracoronary ultrasound imaging devices in the future.

Introduction

In spite of the explosive proliferation of catheter technology over the past 45 years [1–3], there is little published data concerning the mechanical design of such devices. In fact, we are aware of only two reports with quantitative information on catheter stiffness [4, 5]. Recent requirements to apply catheter systems in more inaccessible areas of the body and to perform new diagnostic and therapeutic procedures have led to a greater need for information to predict catheter behavior in vivo.

As an example, the new interest in intracoronary ultrasound imaging devices pose many new design problems. In these devices, not only are there stringent ultrasound considerations, but there are also multiple mechanical and electrical design requirements as well. In this paper, we consider factors that affect the ability of a percutaneous catheter to traverse the tortuous vessel pathways in human coronary artery catheterization. The resultant equations developed are then utilized to predict the force required to overcome the frictional resistance in this passage. Next, the requirements of rotating an ultrasonic transducer at the tip of a catheter in order to generate tomographic images of the vessel wall are considered. Torque requirements and the transmission of the torque to the tip are analyzed with numerical results compiled of both the torque and the resulting twisting action of the catheter body. We then specifically focus on the design of flexible drive cables for transducer rotation. Finally, factors involved in the connection of the ultrasonic transducer to the external electronic processing and display unit are discussed and some numerical results given.

Mechanical considerations

Several factors become apparent when catheterizing an intravascular site. Foremost is the bending and torsional stiffness of the catheter. Its flexural rigidity is responsible for the force it applies to the wall of the vessel as it traverses the tortuous vessel pathway. This force produces a frictional drag which opposes movement or rotation of the catheter. Rotational opposition results in torsional twisting along the catheter. The moduli of the catheter material affect both the amount of force on the vessel wall as well as the amount of torsional twisting that will result. Other considerations are: curvature which may be preformed in the catheter, plastic deformation of the catheter under load, temperature effects, cross sectional geometry, additive wires or cables, and the outer catheter surface characteristics. Finally, the coefficient of friction between the catheter and the wall is of paramount importance. In the discussion that follows, all of these issues cannot be addressed; the reader is referred to Jang [6] for further information.

First, it is helpful to review a few definitions of friction before beginning the analysis. Friction is considered to be the resistance to motion between two objects in contact. Static friction is the friction involved in just starting the motion, whereas kinetic friction is the friction found when an object is moving [7]. Both are of concern in introducing a catheter.

The coefficient of friction, useful in analysis, is defined as the ratio of two forces involved. The numerator of this ratio is the force required to start or maintain motion in a direction tangential to the surface between the two objects. The denominator is the force that is applied normal to this surface by one object on the other. The coefficient has been found to be a constant value in some cases, but often varies with a number of factors. For example, if the surfaces are dry or wet by a lubricating agent, considerable difference exists. If lubricated, the coefficient may be a function of the applied normal force between the objects as well as a function of the velocity of motion of the objects [8]. Temperature and the types of materials involved are other important variables.

Accurate calculations of the forces needed to move a catheter in a blood vessel require knowledge of the coefficient of friction of the catheter against the wall. Unfortunately, published data are scarce. There is a report on the coefficient in friction of suture material [9] and a report on urinary catheters [10], but these are of limited help. In the general engineering literature, the coefficient of friction has been reported for only one biological material (leather), several biological fluids used as lubricants (such as animal fat and whale oil), several polymers, and a variety of solids [7, 8, 11].

In Table 1 relevant coefficients from the literature are presented. The value of the coefficient of friction for Teflon (E.I. du Pont de Nemours Co., Wilmington, Del. trademark for polytetrafluoroethylene) on itself and other materials (.04) represents one of the lowest values of friction obtainable without special lubricants. Therefore, the coefficient of friction of a polymer or metal against the inner wall of a blood vessel, in the presence of blood or saline, is probably greater than this. We can only speculate on actual, in vivo coefficients of friction and measurements will have to be made to provide accurate information.

Derivation of force equations

Catheter advancement can be modeled using well known forces for a small section followed by gener-

Table 1. Coefficients of static friction

Material	Coefficient	Material	Coefficient
Polyethylene on polyethylene	0.2	Leather on metal (dry)	0.6
Polyethylene on steel	0.2	Leather on metal (wet)	0.4
Teflon on Teflon	0.04	Leather on metal (greasy)	0.2
Teflon on steel	0.04	Steel on steel (animal sperm)	0.1
Nylon on nylon	0.15–0.25	Steel on steel (animal lard)	0.085
Steel on steel	0.58	Steel on base white metal (long chain fatty acid)	0.08

alization to the entire catheter. Consider a short catheter section illustrated in Fig. 1A. If a torque (T) is applied to one end while the other is held fixed, the free end will twist through an angle (θ). The equation which describes the relationship between the torque and θ (degrees) is:

$$\theta = 57.3 \; TL/JG \tag{1}$$

where L = length of the catheter held, G = the shear modulus for the catheter material and J = the polar moment of inertia [12, 13]. This moment for a catheter with a single lumen, coaxial in nature, with an outer diameter (d_1) and inner diameter (d_2) is expressed by:

$$J = \pi \; (d_1^4 - d_2^4)/32 \tag{2}$$

More complex catheter cross sections will require a different equation for calculating J. In Fig. 1B, the distance (h) a catheter will bend when a force (F) is applied in a direction normal to the axis of the catheter is illustrated. The relationship between F and h are given by:

$$h = FL^3/3EI \tag{3a}$$

where E = Young's modulus of the catheter material and I = the moment of inertia around a line passing through the center of gravity of a cross section of the catheter. For a single lumen coaxial configuration, I = J/2.

These equations can be used to measure E and G for various materials by loading them with a force F and measuring h to determine E and by applying a torque T and measuring θ to determine G. These measurements have been performed for a number of commonly used catheters and catheter materials [5]. Selected results are summarized in Fig. 2. The importance of assessing the values of moduli at body temperature in contrast to room temperature is apparent in the figure.

Catheter insertion

The forces on the catheter at various places can be

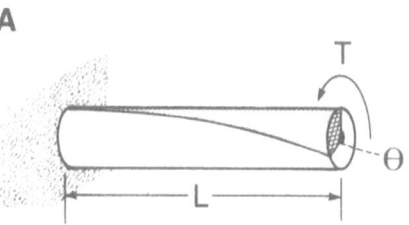

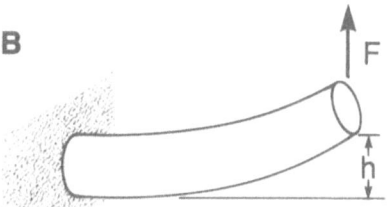

Fig. 1. A section of a catheter mounted as a cantilever beam with applied torque and force. A. The twist angle θ that results from an applied torque is shown. B. The displacement h that results from the transverse force F is illustrated.

piecewise predicted knowing E and I of the catheter if the vessel pathway can be numerically described in three-dimensional space. In Fig. 3A, a catheter is shown lying in a blood vessel. The catheter is bent due to vessel curvature. The catheter's accommodating curvature can be approximated by points along its midline as shown. The points can be chosen as close together as necessary to provide a more accurate description. A set of three points can be used to describe the curvature of the vessel in a subregion (Figs. 3A & B): P_i, P_{i-1} and P_{i-2}. For analysis, points P_{i-2} and P_{i-1} can be considered a straight section and P_i as the point that departs from this straight line. The force F_i perpendicular to this line applied to the catheter at point P_i can be calculated using equation 3 after rearrangement, where h = the normal distance from point P_i to an extended line through P_{i-1} and P_{i-2}.

$$F = 3hEI/L^3 \tag{3b}$$

L in this case is the sum of the distances P_{i-2} to P_{i-1} and P_{i-1} to P_i. The use of this equation assumes that the catheter was initially straight and not pre-curved. The force applied to the catheter results from the curvature forces on it by the blood vessel,

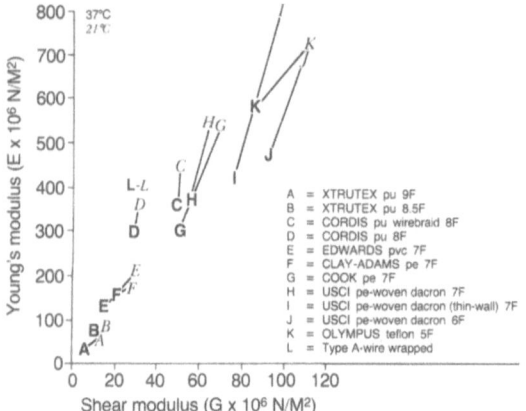

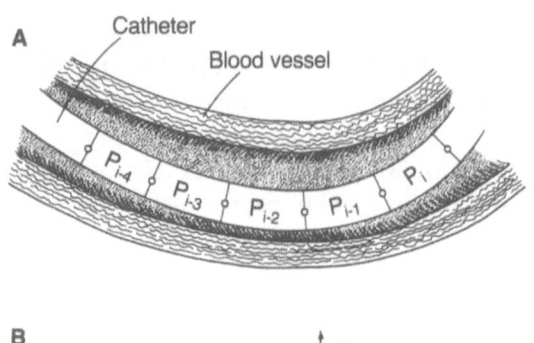

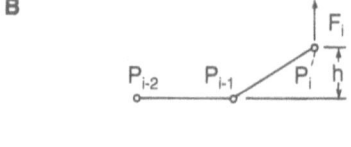

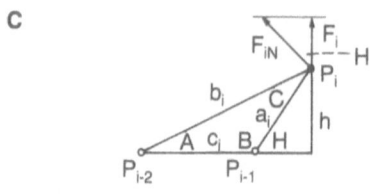

Fig. 2. Moduli values measured at two temperatures (37° C bold and 21° C script letters) for different catheters and catheter material. The manufactures' names are shown in capital letters, pu = polyurethane, pu wirebraid 8F = 8 French pu catheter reinforced with steel wire braid, pvc = polyvinylchloride, pe = polyethylene, pe-woven dacron = pe catheter reinforced with dacron braid, Teflon = polytetrafluoroethylene, and Type A-wire wrapped = pu catheter wrapped with copper wire and coated with Biomer (Ethnor Inc).

the catheter's material modulus and its moment of inertia. The resistive force produced by friction between the catheter and the vessel wall is a key factor in advancing a catheter in a blood vessel. This friction is due to the summation of forces perpendicular to the axis of the catheter times the coefficient of friction between the catheter and the blood vessel wall. For the three points mentioned above in Fig. 3B, the force perpendicular to the axis of the catheter at point P_i need only be in considered, F_{iN} in Fig. 3C. Although in actuality this force is distributed along the P_{i-1} to P_i section, it is assumed to be a lumped force at point P_i. This assumption holds if the points are chosen close to each other. The various angles (A, B, C, & H) and lengths of sides (a_i, b_i, c_i & h) of triangles formed by these points and the projection of P_i onto a straight line formed by P_{i-1} and P_{i-1} are also illustrated. (Note the angles and h are also a function of i, but for simplicity they will not labeled with the subscript i.) From the law of cosines,

$$\cos(A) = (b_i^2 + c_i^2 - a_i^2)/2b_ic_i$$
$$\text{so } A = \cos^{-1}((b_i^2 + c_i^2 - a_i^2)/2b_ic_i) \quad [4]$$

Fig. 3. A. A catheter lying in a blood vessel. Various points are shown in the center line of the catheter which indicate the position of the catheter in three dimensional space. B. Shows the relationship of three points of the catheter and a transverse force F_i and displacement h. C. Details a further elaboration of B. showing the formation of a triangle with the angles and sides labeled.

and for right triangles,

$$\sin(A) = h/b_i \text{ so } h = b_i \sin(A)$$
$$\text{and } \sin(H) = h/a_i \text{ and } H = \sin^{-1}(h/a_i).$$
$$\text{Substituting for h, } H = \sin^{-1}((b_i/a_i) \sin(A)) \quad [5]$$

One can also see in Fig. 3C that the normal force F_{iN} and F_i are related by

$$F_{iN} = F_i/\cos(H) \quad [6]$$

Equations 6, 5, and 4 relate the forces to distance between the points. Each point has a Cartesian coordinate description such that P_i is described in space as (x_i, y_i, z_i). Therefore,

$$a_i = \{ (x_i - x_{i-1})^2 + (y_i - y_{i-1})^2 + (z_i - z_{i-1})^2 \}^{1/2} \quad [7]$$
$$b_i = \{ (x_i - x_{i-2})^2 + (y_i - y_{i-2})^2 + (z_i - z_{i-2})^2 \}^{1/2} \quad [8]$$
$$c_i = \{ (x_{i-1} - x_{i-2})^2 + (y_{i-1} - y_{i-2})^2 + (z_{i-1} - z_{i-2})^2 \}^{1/2}$$
$$[9]$$

Equation 3b can be used to find F_i recognizing that $L = a_i + c_i$:

$$F_i = 3EIh/ (a_i + c_i)^3 \qquad [10]$$

The normal force due to bending (F_{iN}, equation 6) can be calculated given the coordinate values for the three points and E and I for the catheter. The force of friction due to this normal force is then related by the coefficient of friction (C_f) between the catheter and the vessel wall under the lubricating properties of blood or saline, whichever is present. This coefficient may be a constant or a variable. If it is a function of the normal force, then a 'look up' table can be used during numerical calculation to select the appropriate value based on the normal force present. For the remaining discussion, the coefficient will be held constant due to the lack of information about it in blood vessels.

If the catheter is being advanced to the right there will be additional forces on the P_{i-1} to P_i section due to the resisting forces from the section to the right of P_i (Fig. 3A). This force can be considered an axial force, F_{ai} (Fig. 4) which is the force on section P_i to P_{i+1} projected onto an extended line formed by points P_{i-1} and P_i. This force must also be present at point P_{i-1}. For the catheter at point P_{i-1} to be advanced, an axial force, F_{ai-1}, (Fig. 4) must be applied. F_{ai-1} will be the vector sum of the force normal to the axis of section P_{i-1} to P_i (F_{iNa}, Fig. 4) and the sum of the forces along the axis of the section. The forces along the axis will be the sum of the axial force (F_{ai}) and the total frictional force on that section (F_{ift}). It can be seen from the geometry on Fig. 4 that

$$\cos(H) = (F_{ai} + F_{ift})/F_{ai-1} \qquad [11]$$
$$\text{so } F_{ai-1} = (F_{ai} + F_{ift})/ \cos(H)$$

Summing all the normal forces to the section P_{i-1} to P_1 (see Fig. 4) and multiplying by the coefficient of friction gives the total frictional force on this section:

$$F_{ift} = C_f(F_{iNa} + F_{iN}). \qquad [12]$$

From Fig. 4, $\sin(H) = F_{iNa} / F_{ai-1}$

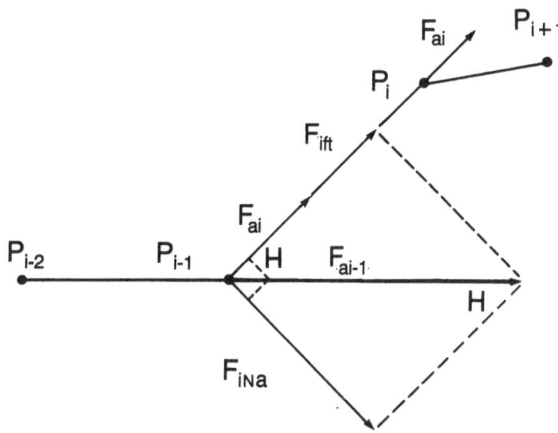

Fig. 4. Illustration and labeling of the additional forces that occur on the subsection of Fig. 3C when the catheter is being advanced.

so $F_{ift} = C_f(F_{ai-1} \sin(H) + F_{iN}).$

Substituting into equation 11,

$$F_{ai-1} = (F_{ai} + C_fF_{ai-1}\sin(H) + C_fF_{iN})/\cos(H),$$

and separating F_{ai-1} produces:

$$F_{ai-1} (1 - C_f \tan(H)) = (F_{ai} + C_fF_{iN})/\cos(H) \qquad [13]$$

which reduces to:

$$F_{ai-1} = (F_{ai} + C_fF_{iN})/(\cos(H) - C_f \sin(H)). \qquad [14]$$

Therefore, when calculating equation 14, F_{ai} from the section to the right of P_i is used, the coordinates of P_{i-2}, P_{i-1} and P_i are applied to it in equations 7, 8, and 9 to determine a_1, b_i, and c_i and then they in turn are used in equations 4, 5, and 6 to find A, H, and F_{iN}. Equation 14 then determines the axial force at point P_{i-1} to move the catheter to the right. This equation can be iteratively applied by decreasing the index, i, where i = 1, 2, ...n, from n (the point where the tip is located) toward the point where the catheter enters the body. The summation is stopped at i = 3 because of the way the three points P_i, P_{i-1}, and P_{i-2} of the subregion are defined.

Catheter rotation

Two conditions of the catheter are of interest: (a) when the longitudinal position of the catheter in the vessel is stationary and (b) when the catheter is being advanced along the vessel. The torque required to rotate the catheter in these cases as well as the amount of twist that occurs in the catheter between the vessel entrance site and the tip of the catheter are important. Both the catheter resisting torque and the twisting angle are due to the friction of the catheter on the vessel wall. We assume for simplicity that the rotational coefficient of friction is the same as the longitudinal translation coefficient of friction. The solution for the subregion defined by points P_{i-2} to P_i is derived, followed by an extension to a solution for the entire catheter.

The frictional force for the stationary catheter is only due to F_{iN}. The resistive torque, as shown in Fig. 5, will be T_{is} which is assumed for simplicity to be a lumped torque occurring at P_i. The radius of the catheter is the moment arm through which the friction acts, so the describing equation for the torque is:

$$T_{is} = (d_1/2)\, C_f\, F_{iN}. \qquad [15]$$

where d_1 = the outer diameter of the catheter. Applying this formula to equation 1 and using $J = 2I$ for the single lumen coaxial catheter gives the twisting angle (θ_{is}) that occurs in the P_{i-1} to P_i section:

$$\theta_{is} = 28.65\, a_i\, T_{is}/GI \qquad [16]$$

where a_i = the distance between P_{i-1} and P_i (equation 7).

The total torque (T_{ts}) required to rotate the catheter and the resulting total twist (θ_{ts}) when the tip to the catheter is at position P_n is:

$$T_{ts} = \sum_{i=n}^{3} T_{is} \qquad [17]$$

$$\text{and } \theta_{ts} = \sum_{i=n}^{3} \theta_{is} = (28.65 / GI) \sum_{i=n}^{3} a_i\, T_{is} \qquad [18]$$

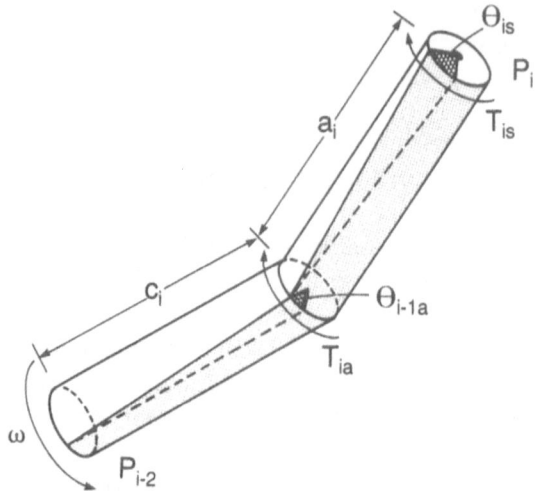

Fig. 5. The torque and twist angles that result on a subsection when a catheter is being rotated at a velocity ω. This is the subsection for points P_i, P_{i-1}, and P_{i-2} as shown in Fig. 3.

When the catheter is being advanced there is an additional normal force applied to the catheter in the subregion, F_{iNa}, which we assume is applied at P_{i-1} (Fig. 4). The result is an additive, resisting frictional torque (T_{ia}), which produces a twisting deflection along the P_{i-2} to P_{i-1} section (Fig. 5, θ_{i-1a}). The equations are:

$$T_{ia} = (d_1/2)\, C_f\, F_{iNa} = (d_1/2)\, C_f\, F_{ai-1}\sin(H) \qquad [19]$$

$$\text{and } \theta_{i-1a} = (28.65\, c_i/GI)\, T_{ia} \qquad [20]$$

where c_i is the length shown in Fig. 3C. The total torque in this case (T_{tav}) is

$$T_{tav} = \sum_{i=n}^{3} (T_{ia} + T_{is}) \qquad [21]$$

The total angle of deflection will be the summation of the deflections produced by equations 18 and 20:

$$\theta_{tav} = \theta_{ts} + \sum_{i=n}^{3} \theta_{i-1a} =$$

$$(28.65/GI) \sum_{i=n}^{3} (a_i T_{is} + c_i T_{isa}) \qquad [22]$$

Therefore, the rotational torque and twisting angles are respectively given by the equations 17 & 18 for the stationary catheter and equations 21 & 22 for the advancing catheter.

Flexible drive cables

Generating a cross sectional ultrasonic image of the blood vessel wall from a catheter requires spatial rotation of an ultrasonic beam circumferentially around the catheter. This may be accomplished electronically [14] or by mechanically rotating a single transducer element. We consider the latter approach in this discussion. One of the key concerns is the method of coupling rotational drive force to the transducer located at the catheter tip. As mentioned earlier, Young's modulus of the catheter affects the rotational drag and the resulting twisting angle between the tip and the entrance site of the catheter. Similarly, a drive cable located in the catheter for rotating the transducer will have rotational friction and a non zero twisting angle. The magnitude of this friction and twisting angle will depend on the vessel curvature, as well as catheter insertion distance. Low rotational friction and low or at least unvarying twist angle is desirable to provide smooth rotation of the scanning transducer and to maintain registration between the transducer's positional angle and the electronic angle tracking circuitry. Furthermore, to minimize twisting angle (θ), the shear modulus (G) for the drive shaft should be high (see Equation 1). Hence it becomes apparent that a low value of E and a high value of G are desirable. Fig. 2 shows the relations between E and G we found for many plastics. For metals and other homogenous solids operating in the elastic region, E and G are related by Poisson's ratio (μ), $E = 2(1 + \mu)G$, where $\mu =$ lateral strain/longitudinal strain. For E to be less than G, μ would have to be negative. We therefore need a cable that is not homogenous.

A cable has been constructed (Baird Industries, Ho-Ho-Kus, New Jersey) with these properties. It is included in a small imaging probe used with an endoscope for imaging the gastrointestinal wall [15–17]. Construction of this drive cable is shown in Fig. 6. It is composed of three counterwound layers

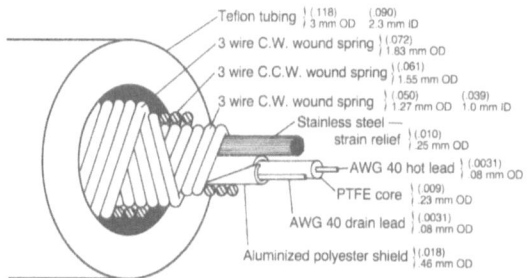

Fig. 6. A catheter design shown which has been used for endoscopic ultrasound. The catheter includes a flexibe cable composed of three layers of alternately wound steel wire. An electrical cable is included inside of the inner-most layer for connecting to the transducer.

of 3 parallel spring steel wires of 0.135 mm diameter. In Fig. 7A, the manner in which parallel windings are applied to a cable is illustrated. The cable, illustrated in Fig. 6, is extremely flexible in the lateral direction and yet has excellent torsional characteristics. For example, the cable itself without the outer Teflon sheath (Fig. 6) can be wrapped around the index finger three times and be easily rotated with applied torque that is less than 7×10^{-4} N-m. The moduli values measured for this cable were: $E = 11.45 \times 10^6$ N/m^2 and $G = 139 \times 10^6$ N/m^2.

The high torsional rigidity of this cable is due to its multilayered counter-wound construction. These counter-wound layers expand or contract depending on the direction they are wound with respect to the direction of rotation. Since the direction of winding is alternated for each layer, expansion and contraction occurs alternately between the layers. This action makes them bind together, thereby increasing the cable's total shear modulus. Note, that if the cable is to be rotated in clockwise and counter clockwise directions at various times, then three layers are required for proper binding action. However, if the cable is rotated in only one direction, then only two layers are needed. This principal of obtaining high torsional rigidity is illustrated in Fig. 7B for a two layer counter wound cable. The lateral flexibility remains very low for this design of cable because laterally it still acts as two helical springs. The use of several parallel

A

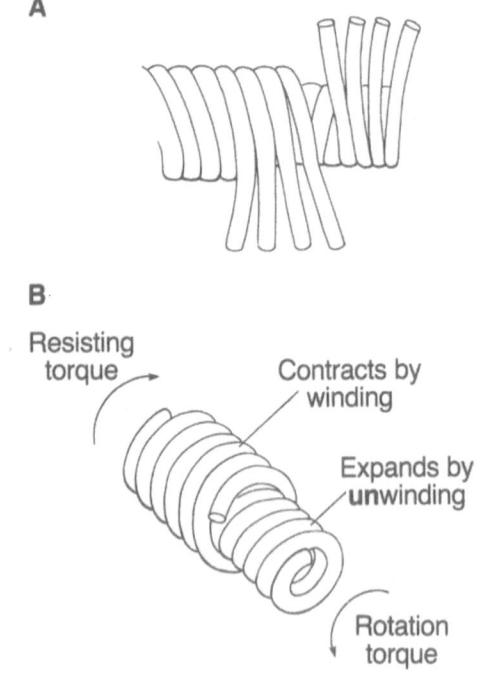

B

Resisting torque

Contracts by winding

Expands by **un**winding

Rotation torque

Fig. 7. Two layer helically wound coaxial drive cable. A. The method in which several parallel wires may be used to wind layers of the cable. B. The manner in which two layers bind together to increase the torsional rigidity. The outer layer contracts and inner layer expands when torque is applied in the direction illustrated.

wires wound together (as illustrated in Fig. 7A), in contrast to a single wire, is a method that has been employed for a considerable time in making flexible drive cables [18]. The greater the number of parallel wires, the greater is the pitch of each individual helical coil in the cable. Increasing the pitch this way increases the lateral flexibility of the cable [19]. However, theoretical and experimental work are needed to develop equations that will predict more exactly the characteristics of this type of drive cable.

Use of catheter pathways to calculate forces, torques and torsion angles

The above equations were applied to the problem of Judkins (transfemoral) coronary catheterization. A program was written in a general high level language designed specifically for scientific calculations (PCMATLAB, the MathWorks, Inc., Sherborn, MA) to calculate the forces, torques, and twist angles. This program was used on an IBM AT equivalent computer with a coprocessor (80287, Intel Corp., Santa Clara, CA). The program as well as blood vessel positional information is available from the authors on request. The numerical description of x, y, z positions along the femoral artery and aorta were acquired from a cross sectional anatomy text [20]. The distance from the back of the cadaver slice to the artery and the lateral distance from the midline were measured from the pictures provided in the text. Longitudinal position of the vessel was determined by multiplying the cross sectional number from the beginning slice by 1.3 cm, the depth of each individual cut. Measurements were performed from sections beginning at the level of the superior portion of the symphysis pubis (longitudinal position considered to be 0) and extending to the superior region of the aortic arch. At the beginning level, the femoral artery is close to the surface of the skin, providing the standard cannulation site for Judkins (transfemoral) catheterization [1].

The cross sections were from two male cadavers, with sections overlapping at the T12 spinal level. These overlapping regions were used to adjust the rest of the cross sections to allow approximation of a single subject. Since there is no scaling given with regard to the dimensions of the cross sectional images they are assumed to be of equal scale. The dimensions were scaled so that the width at the mid chest region was equal in value to the chest of one of the authors. Finally, since the individual cross sections do not reflect the arch of the back, we compensated for this again using measurements from ourselves. The data was then smoothed with three point averaging in each direction.

The anatomical positions of the coronary arteries were obtained from the work of Dodge and associates [21]. In their report they determined the three dimensional position of the coronary arteries from biplane angiography and referenced them with respect to the left main coronary ostium. Their data were taken from 37 patients; the subset of data we used, were the averages from 19 right coronary dominant men. The beginning position for each coronary artery from their work was added to the ending point in the ascending aorta. This action allowed us to describe the complete pathway of transfemoral coronary catheterization.

The numerical values for the position of the arteries were all converted and expressed in Cartesian coordinates following the definitions of Dodge et al. [21] where x = the lateral distance from midline with the subject's left representing the positive direction, y representing the longitudinal position with the increasing positive value in the superior or cranial direction, and z representing the posterior to anterior direction with increasing positive values in the anterior direction. The origin for z was chosen at the posterior of the cross section acquired at the first level, the catheterization site. Fig 8 shows this data and illustrates the catheter pathways from the femoral artery to the left anterior descending (LAD), left circumflex (LCx), and right coronary (RGA) arteries. The coronary artery termination points used for this plot were: L_4 — the LAD wrap around segment, C4 — the LCx distal circumflex just proximal to the posterior wall branch and R_4 — the left ventricular extension branch. The y axis is the ordinate axis in this figure.

Calculations of force, torque, and twisting angle using these positional data are plotted in Figs. 9–12. In Fig. 9, four curves are shown. Two are for a polyethylene catheter studied at two coefficient of friction values. The second pair are for a flexible drive cable (made of helical steel wire as illustrated in Fig. 7), also studied at these same coefficient of friction values. Both catheter and cable are coaxial in nature with an outer diameter of 1.43 mm and inner diameter of 1.0 mm, a typical size used in coronary artery catheters. All the calculations (Figs. 9–13) were made with these dimensions and using the following moduli: $E = 156.8 \times 10^6$ N/m^2 and $G = 14.0 \times 10^6$ N/m^2 for polyethylene at body temperature and $E = 11.45 \times 10^6$ N/m^2 and $G = 139 \times 10^6$ N/m^2 for the flexible drive cable (These values were measured for a cable of the design illustrated in Fig. 6). The coefficients of friction in our calculations were chosen to approximate the range of friction encountered in normal catheterization. The value of 0.04 represents Teflon on

Teflon or Teflon on steel. The inner lumen of many femoral to coronary guide catheters are coated with Teflon, so this may represent a real value for a flexible drive cable inside such a catheter. Most likely the coefficient of any catheter material on a blood vessel wall is probably greater than $C_f = 0.04$; therefore, this value is low for the overall length of femoral to the distal region of the coronary artery. The other coefficient used, $C_f = 0.2$, is a value for polyethylene on polyethylene without lubricant. This value does not represent the highest value of friction one can encounter with various materials, but may approximate the highest practical value since the surfaces of catheters or drive cables will most likely be lubricated by saline, plasma or other substances.

The differences in results between the flexible cable and the polyethylene cable and the two values of coefficients of friction are quite apparent in Figs. 9 and 10. The advantage of the flexible cable design for rotating a transducer is striking. The graph at the right side of Fig. 9 is the case in which the catheter is being rotated and advanced. The rotational torque was found to be considerably less for the case of a stationary catheter, but is not shown here for simplicity. However, in Fig. 10 the rotational twist angle is shown for both cases. Clearly the twist angle will vary significantly as one begins to advance the catheter from a stationary point for the polyethylene catheter and the flexible cable with $C_f = 0.2$, particularly if the tip is well into the LAD. In Figs. 11 and 12 similar values of forces, torques and twist angles are shown for catheterization of the RCA and the LCx. For simplicity, the calculations in these later graphs are only for the flexible cable and the higher value of C_f, 0.2.

Electrical wire for connecting the transducer

The electrical connection to the transducer is a particularly important part of designing a scanning ultrasonic catheter. There are at least seven major considerations. These are cable: (a) size, (b) flexibility, (c) durability, (d) characteristic impedance, (e) shielding, (f) electrical transmission loss, and (g) purchasing cost. Many of these requirements are in conflict with each other.

210

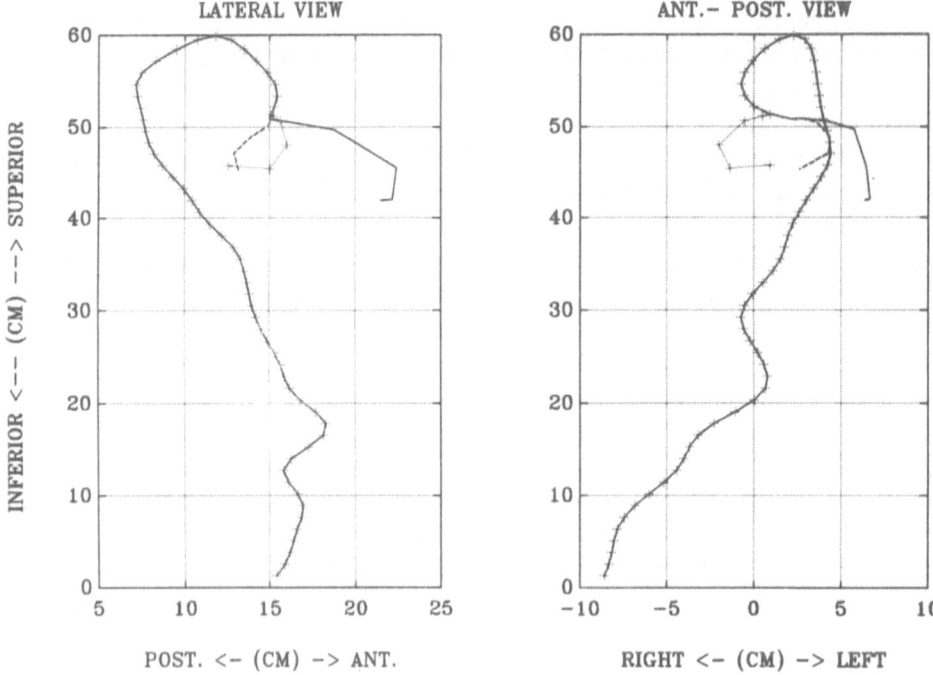

Fig. 8. Two views of the transfemoral pathway of a catheter: solid line – left anterior descending (through L4 middle branch), dashed line – left circumflex (through the C4 middle branch), and dot and plus – the right coronary artery (through the R4 middle branch). ANT. – POST. = anterior – posterior.

One of the authors has employed three different wire configurations in various miniature ultrasonic probes. The most elegant and costly type is a microcoax with 0.203 mm (0.008″) outside diameter and 50 Ω characteristic impedance [22]. Two styles were used, UT-8 and UT-8S, both manufactured by Micro-coax Components, Inc., Collegeville, PA. The outer coating is a thin-wall, rigid tube composed of copper for UT-8 and silver for UT-8S. The copper type was found to break easily when flexed several times through sharp angles, whereas the silver is much more resilient and durable. The copper type is less expensive but the cost of either would be a major problem in disposable or short life ultrasonic catheters. A second microcoax (Gore and Associates, Huntington Beach, CA, model CXN-1562) that we have used [15–17, 23] is illustrated in Fig. 6. It is much less expensive, offers 50 Ω characteristic impedance and tolerates flexing very well. However, its diameter is much larger, 0.46 mm (0.018″) and we are uncertain whether a smaller diameter cable can be fabricated. Simple

wire pairs, individually insulated and bonded together, have been used. They offer a consistent characteristic impedance (50Ω nominally), are flexible, and low in cost. One source for such wire is MWS Wire Industries, Westlake Village, CA. Their multifilar model B2362111 consists of two 36 gauge copper wires insulated with polyurethane. A problem with this type of cable is its lack of shielding, making it more susceptible to radio frequency interference.

We have learned that in order to minimize breakage within the catheter, the design must allow sufficient wire slack during extreme catheter bending. An alternative approach is to spiral the cable down the catheter. This method minimizes wire stress with flexing while avoiding additional catheter stiffness due to the wire. In Fig. 2, catheter L was made by spiraling 32 gage copper wire at a pitch length of 4 mm around catheter material identical to A in the figure. Note that the values of E and G increased. If the cable is a pair of wires as mentioned above, and they are spiraled together,

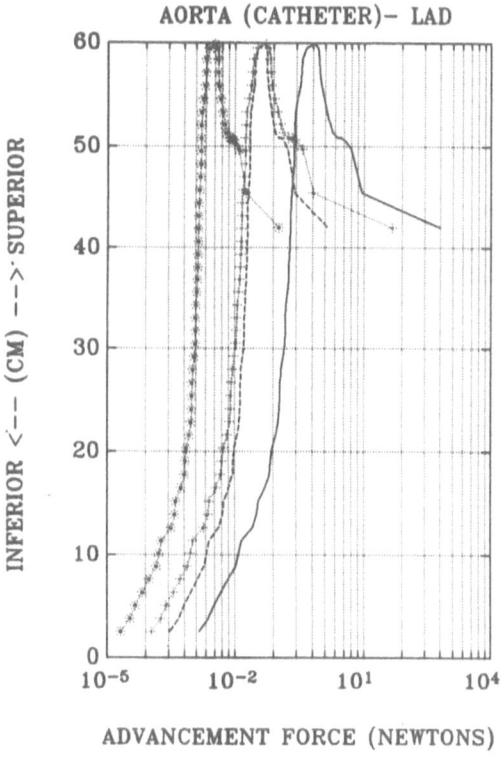
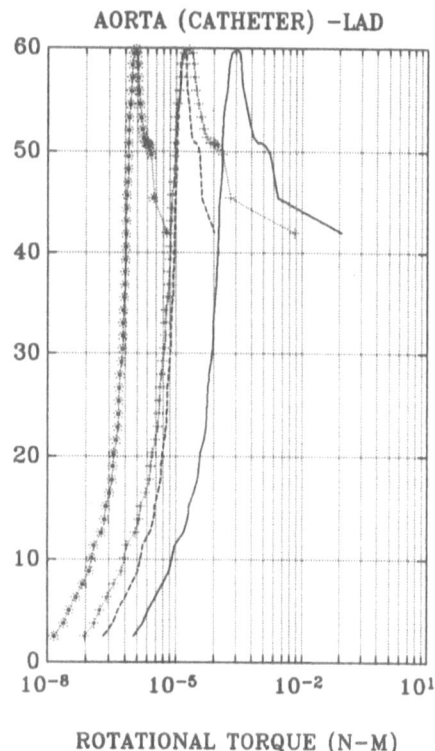

Fig. 9. Advancement force and rotational torque calculated for a catheter or cable being passed transfemorally into the left anterior descending (LAD) coronary artery. (See Fig. 8 to relate an ordinate position to lateral and anterior-posterior positions in the vessel.) The torques shown in the right graph were computed for a catheter being advanced into the vessel. The lines: solid – polyethylene catheter with $C_f = 0.2$, dashed – polyethylene catheter with $C_f = 0.04$, dotted and plus – a flexible drive cable with $C_f = 0.2$, and dot and asterisks – a flexible drive cable with $C_f = 0.04$.

then there is no effect on the characteristic impedance. On the other hand, if only one wire is spiraled and the other is not, the spiraled wire becomes a series inductor and interferes with transmission.

Finally, it may be feasible to include the wire as part of the helically spiraled wire composing the flexible drive cable. The pitch of the spiraling becomes very important for small wire in this case because if the pitch is small then the length of the wire required for fabrication can be surprisingly long. For small diameter wire, a long length can have a significant resistance, introducing remarkable distributed loss and impedance mismatch between the transceiver and the transducer. This loss may be even greater at the high frequencies used for intravascular imaging.

The equation for the length of single wire required in a cable (Fig. 7A) can be derived by con-

sidering the length of each wrap as equal to the hypotenuse of a right triangle where one side is given by the circumference of the coil and the other by the pitch:

$$L_w = (L_c/p) ((\pi d_c)^2 + p^2)^{1/2} \qquad [23]$$

where L_w = the length of the single wire in the cable, L_c = the length of the cable, d_c = the diameter of the helical coil of the cable as defined as the distance between the center of the wires on opposite sides of the coil, and p = the pitch of the windings. The pitch for tightly wound coils = $N_w d_w$ where N_w = the number of parallel wires wound together and d_w = the diameter of the conducting wire with insulation chosen to be equal to the diameter of the steel wire in the cable it replaces. The electrical resistance of a single wire (R_t) wound as

212

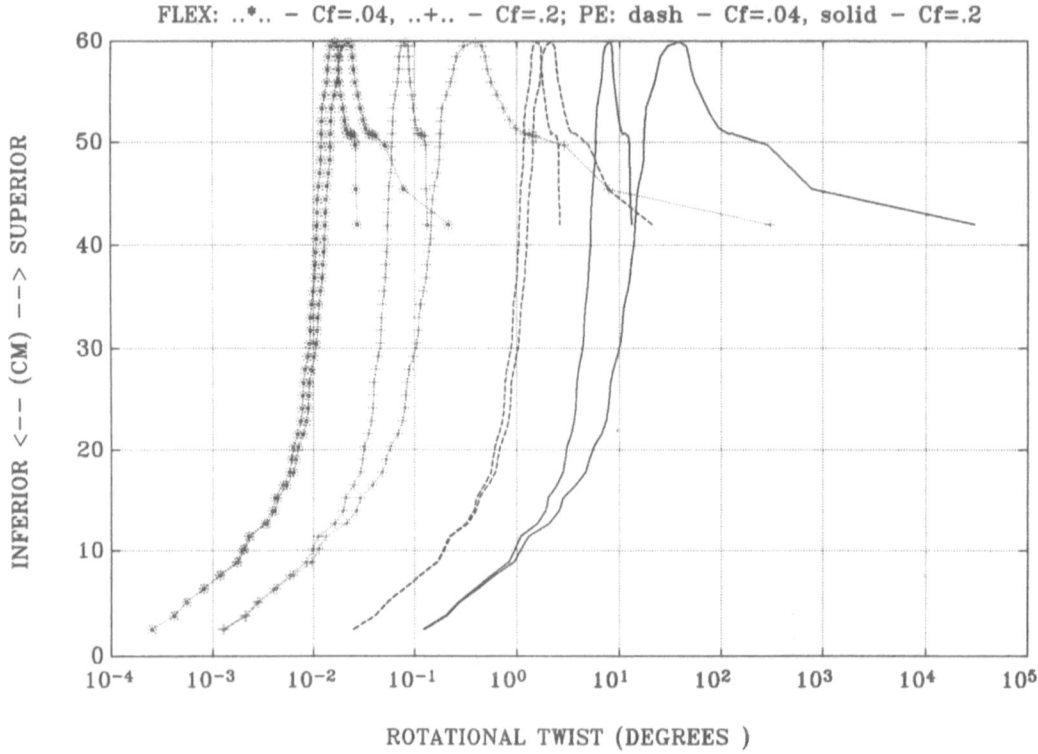

Fig. 10. Rotational twist at various longitudinal positions from the femoral artery to the distal region of the left anterior descending coronary for the flexible cable and a polyethylene catheter. (See Fig. 8 to relate an ordinate location to the respective lateral and anterior-posterior position in the vessel.) Each pair of curves represents both the angle when the catheter is being rotated and advanced (the curve with the greater twist angles) and when it is being rotated with the catheter at a stationary position in the vessel (the curve with the lesser angles). Two values for the coefficient of friction were used in calculation for each case (Cf = 0.04 and 0.2). Nomenclature: FLEX = flexible wire wound cable and PE = polyethylene, dot-asteriks = FLEX at C_f = 0.04, dot-plus = FLEX at C_f = 0.2, dashed = PE at C_f = 0.04 and solid = PE at C_f = 0.2.

one of the parallel wires is given by: $R_t = \varrho L_w/(\pi d^2/4)$ where ϱ = the resistivity of the conductor and d = the diameter of the conductor. Substituting the above equations into this equation provides the following equation for R_t:

$$R_t = (4\varrho L_c/N_w \pi d_w d^2) ((\pi d_c)^2 + (N_w d_w)^2)^{1/2} \quad [24]$$

The resistivity of copper is $1.72 \times 10\text{-}6$ Ω-cm. Calculations for copper for various values of d_w, lengths, and radius N_w are shown in Fig. 13. The insulation thickness for the conductor wire was $25.4\,\mu$m. The high resistance for a cable composed only of a single conductor (ie. no other parallel wires are wrapped with it) is obvious (N = 1 in the left graph). There is a significant decrease in resistance by adding a few wires in parallel (eg. N = 2–5, left graph), but the improvement is less dramatic for larger numbers of wires in parallel (eg. N = 6–10, right graph).

Discussion

The increasing use of catheter-based technology mandates better methods to design catheter devices and predict their behavior in vivo. In this paper, several factors involved in the successful design of a catheter system were described. Equations were developed to predict frictional forces at a single point in a blood vessel, followed by generalization to other points along the vessel. Similarly,

213

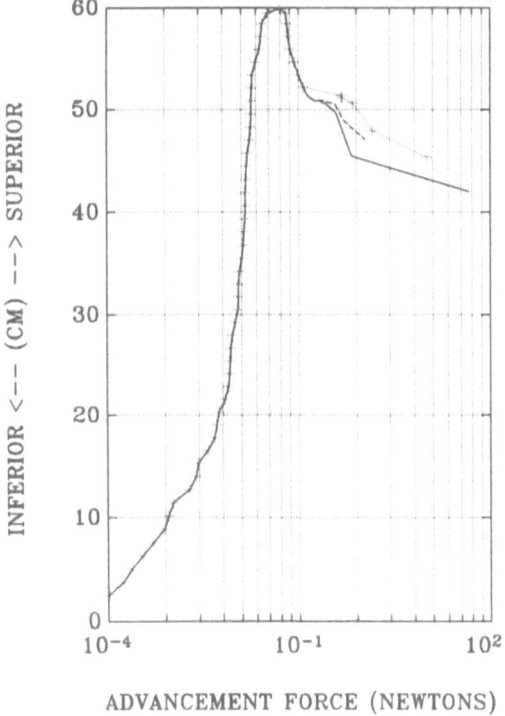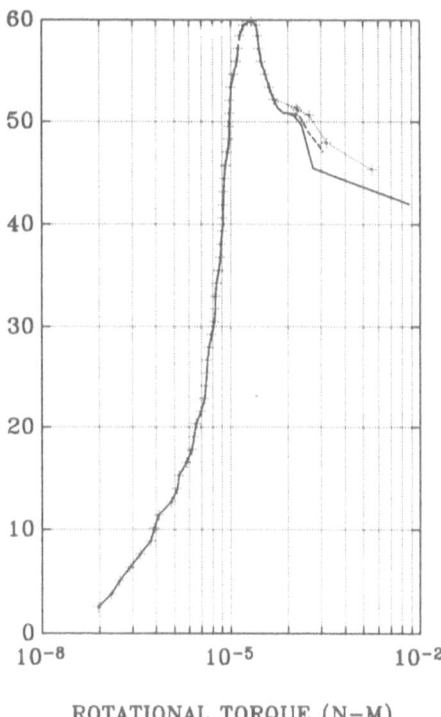

Fig. 11. Flexible cable ($C_f = 0.2$) advancement force and rotational torque at various catheter positions when catheterizing the three coronary arteries: solid – left anterior descending, dashed – left circumflex and dot-plus – right coronary. The ordinate axis represents the distance the catheter has advanced from the catheterization site in the longitudinal direction of the subject. Compare an ordinate point on the graph to Fig. 8 to determine what the lateral and anterior-posterior position is of this point in the vessel.

equations were developed to predict rotational torque and twist angles. These were used to study the feasibility of rotating an ultrasound transducer at the tip of a catheter. A helically spiraled drive cable was shown to be very promising for this purpose. With its high torsional rigidity and low bending stiffness, it minimized the advancement force, rotational torsion and twist angle involved. Such a drive cable offers the possibility of rotating a transducer while allowing external electronic tracking. Little misregistration is predicted between the catheterization entrance to the body and the tip of the device in the vessel, even during advancement. However, high coefficients of friction must be avoided to accomplish this successfully. Incorporating the conductive wire into the windings of such a cable may also be possible if several parallel steel and copper wires are used together in its construction. This may make the design of very small diameter ultrasonic imaging catheters feasible.

There are limitations and approximations to our approach which we will mention. Our analysis and calculations were made with first order approximations. For example, we assumed forces and torques were lump values applied at a particular point in each subregion. An improved approach might consider forces distributed throughout the subregion. Improvements in the method used to identify the location of the femoral – aortic vessel locations would add to the accuracy, as would a finer point location of the position of the coronary arteries. More extensive studies using CAT or MR images of the living are indicated. However, for our first order approximatation, these measurements were adequate since there is considerable variance between people and with posture. Inclusion of worst case analysis for the population variance would also be useful as would the addition of other catheterization sites. We assumed the vessel was much larger than the catheter and the forces applied to it

214

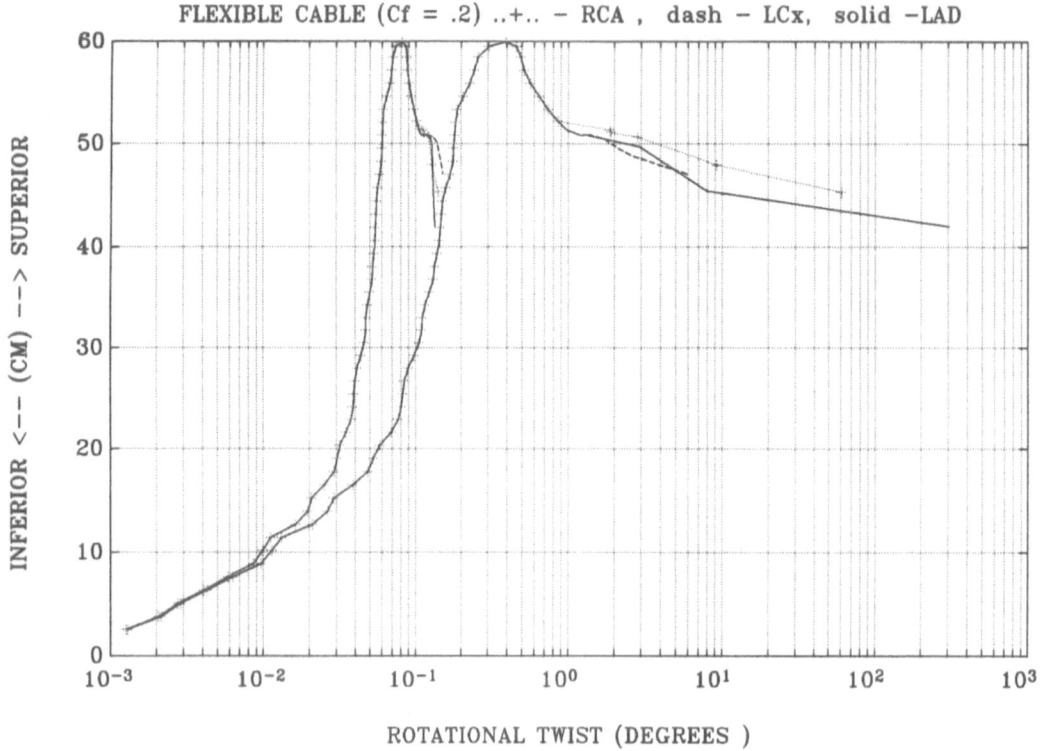

FLEXIBLE CABLE (Cf = .2) ..+.. – RCA , dash – LCx, solid –LAD

Fig. 12. Twist angle between the tip of the catheter and the femoral artery entrance at various positions. Nomenclature for coronary arteries: RCA = right coronary, LCx = left circumflex, and LAD = left anterior descending. These curves were computed for an advancing and rotating flexible cable at $C_f = 0.2$.

were only due to its curvature. No attempt was made to account for extra forces when passing through a tight lesion; study of this aspect of the problem is important but beyond the scope of this paper. The need for experimental data for the coefficients of friction is apparent, because we lacked this information we made estimates of what the values might be. Finally, we have not compared or tested our calculations against experimental data; this will be work for the future.

However, in spite of these concerns our results do parallel clinical observations. The data of Fig. 11 (advancement force and rotational torque versus location) predicts difficulty in distal coronary vessels such as the apical LAD. These data are borne out in clinical coronary angioplasty, where success rates for distal coronary lesions are diminished. Similar analyses would be most useful for comparing catheters composed and coated with various materials and offering various maneuvering char-

acteristics. In addition, these equations could be utilized prospectively to predict mechanical success in reaching a lesion with an angioplasty (or ultrasound) catheter.

To summarize, several numerical methods were described to predict the behavior of both fixed and rotational catheter systems inside blood vessels. These methods have high potential in the design of innovative new catheters. This work strongly supports the theoretical feasibility of building a catheter-based, rotating ultrasound transducer system for coronary artery use.

Acknowledgement

This work was supported by NIH Grants RR04528, HL41464 and DK34814. Dr. Johnson was supported by the American Heart Association, Washington State Affiliate. We thank Robert Mitchell of

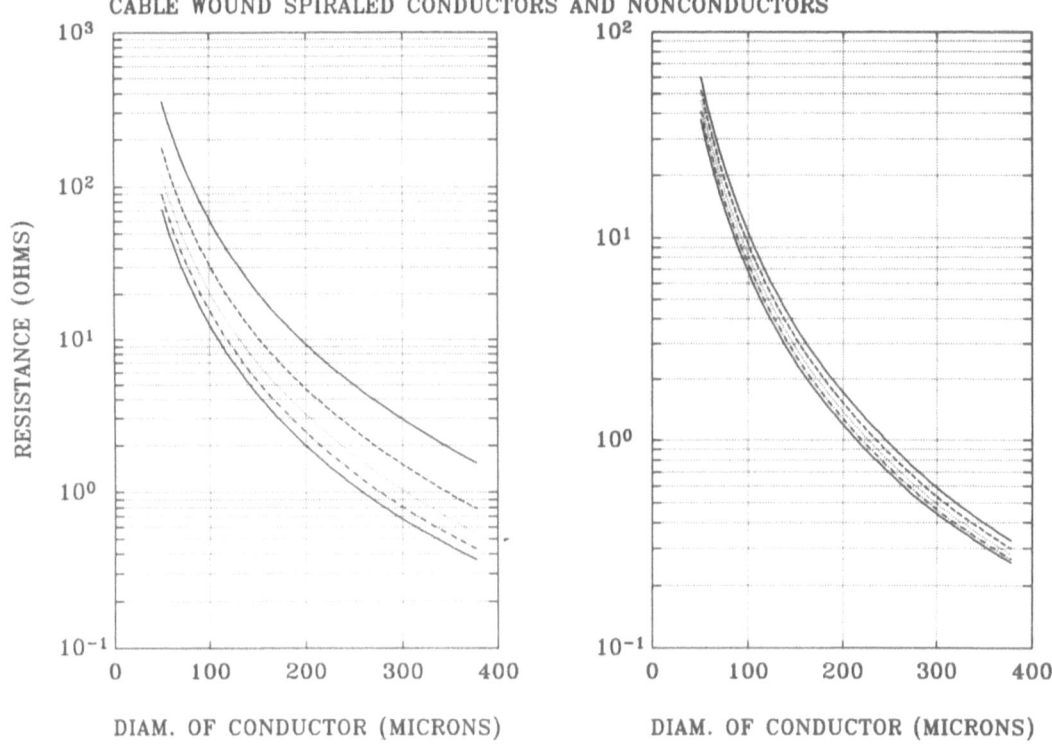

Fig. 13. The resistance versus diameter of copper wire conductor for a 135 cm length flexible cable (1.43 mm OD). The conductive wire is substituted for a steel wire normally used in the cable. The results are for cables with a different number of parallel wires (see Fig. 7A), but with only 1 copper wire substituted. The number of parallel wires used for each curve are progressively 1–5 left graph and 6–10 right graph. Respectively, the number of wires for each designated plotted line are: for the left graph (1 – upper solid, 2 – dashed, 3 – dot, 4 – dash-dot, and 5 – lower solid) and lines for the right graph (6 – upper solid, 7 – dashed, 8 – dot, 9 – dash-dot and 10 – lower solid).

Baird Industries for his creative input and helpful information on the design and fabriction of flexible drive cables.

References

1. Grossman W. Cardiac Catheterization and Angiography, Lea and Febiger, Philadelphia 1980.
2. Cournand A. Cardiac catheterization: Development of the technique, its contributions to experimental medicine, and its initial applications in man. Acta Medica Scandinavica 1975; Supp. 579: 1–32.
3. Zimmerman HA. Intravascular Catheterization. Charles C. Thomas, Springfield, Ill, 1966.
4. Stenquist Q, Curelaru I, Lindner E, Gustavson B. Stiffness of central venous catheters. Acta Anaesthesiol Scand 1983; 27: 153–157.
5. Martin RW, Johnson CC. Engineering considerations of catheters for intravascular ultrasonic measurements. SPIE

Proceedings, Microsensors and Catheter Based Sensing 1989 (in press).
6. Jang DG. Angioplasty, McGraw Hill Book Co., New York 1986.
7. Bowden FP, Tabor D. Friction and Lubrication, Methuen & Co. Ltd., London 1956.
8. Booser RE [ed]. CRC Handbook of Lubrication: Theory and Practice of Tribology, CRC Press, Inc., Boca Raton, Florida, pp. 47, 468, 632, & 643 1984.
9. Gupta BS, Wolf KW, Postlethwait RW. Effect of suture material and construction on frictional properties of sutures. Surgery, Gynecology & Obstertrics. 1985; 161: 12–16.
10. Nickel JC, Olson ME, Costerton JW. In vivo coefficient of kinetic friction: study of urinary catheter biocompatibility. Urology 1987; 29: 501–503.
11. Bowden FP, Tabor D. The Friction and Lubrication of Solids: Appendix X, Some typical values of friction – Metal Surfaces – Unlubricated, ed. by Fowler RH, Kapitza P, Mott NF, Bullard EC, Oxford University Press, pp. 322, 1954.

12. Souders M. The Engineer's Companion: A Concise Handbook of Engineering Fundamentals, John Wiley and Sons, Inc. New York pp. 102–31: 1966.

13. Higdon A, Ohlsen EH, Stiles WB. Mechanics of Materials, John Wiley & Sons, Inc. New York, NY, p. 486, 1960.

14. Bom N, Lancee CT, Egmond FC. An ultrasonic intracardiac scanner. Ultrasonics 1972; 10: 72–6.

15. Martin RW, Silverstein FE, Kimmey MB, Jiranek G, Proctor A. B mode imaging and Doppler ultrasonic catheters for use with fiber optic endoscopes. SPIE Proceedings, Microsensors and Catheter Based Imaging Technology 1988; 904: 121–6.

16. Martin RW, Silverstein FE, Kimmey MB. A 20 MHz ultrasound system for imaging the intestinal wall. Ultrasound Med Biol 1989 (in press).

17. Silverstein FE, Martin RW, Kimmey MB, Jiranek GC, Franklin DW, Proctor A. Experimental evaluation of an endoscopic ultrasound probe: in vitro and in vivo canine studies. Gastroenterology 1989; 96: 1058–62.

18. Rotary Motion Flexible Shafts, Technical Bulletin, S.S. White Industrial Products, Penwalt, 151 Old New Brunswick Road, PO Box 68, Piscataway, NJ.

19. Personal Communication. Mitchell R, Baird Industries, Ho-Ho-Kus, New Jersey 1989.

20. Bo WJ, Meschan I, Krueger WA. Basic Atlas of Cross Sectional Anatomy, W.B. Saunders Company, Philadelphia, PA, pp. 76–186, 1980.

21. Dodge JT, Brown BG, Bolson EL, Dodge HT. Intrathoracic spatial location of specified coronary segments on the normal human heart. Applications in quantitative arteriography, assessment of regional risk and contraction, and anatomic display. Circulation 1988; 78: 1167–80.

22. Martin RW, Watkins DW. An ultrasonic catheter for intravascular measurement of blood flow: Technical details, IEEE Sonics and Ultrasonics, 1980; SV-27: 227–86.

23. Martin RW, Gilbert DA, Silverstein FE, Deltenre M, Tytgat G, Gange RK, Myers J. An endoscopic Doppler probe for assessing intestinal vasculature. Ultrasound Med. Biol. 1985; 11: 61–9.

List of first authors

H. Thomas Aretz, M.D.
Lahey Clinic Medical Center
41 Mall Road
BURLINGTON, MA 01805, U.S.A.

Prof. A.E. Becker, M.D.
Academisch Medisch Centrum
Pathologie H2-134
Meibergdreef 9
NL-1105 AZ, AMSTERDAM

Prof. N. Bom, Ph.D.
Erasmus University Rotterdam
Thoraxcentre, Ee 2302b
P.O. Box 1738
NL-3000 DR, ROTTERDAM

Prof. C. Borst, M.D.
University Hospital Utrecht
Exp. Cardiology
Mail stop 62002
Catharijnesingel 101
NL-3511 GV, UTRECHT

R.J. Crowley, B.Sc.
Boston Scientific Corp.
480 Pleasant Street
WATERTOWN, MA 02172, U.S.A.

W.J. Gussenhoven, M.D.
Erasmus University Rotterdam
Thoraxcentre, Ee 2302
P.O. Box 1738
NL-3000 DR, ROTTERDAM

Craig J. Hartley, Ph.D.
Section Cardiovascular Sciences
Baylor College of Medicine
One Baylor Plaza
Texas Medical Center
HOUSTON, TX 77030, U.S.A.

John McB. Hodgson, M.D.
Cardiac Catheterization Lab
Hunter Holmes McGuire
Medical Center
1201 Broad Rock Boulevard
RICHMOND, VA 23249, U.S.A.

Richard E. Kerber, M.D.
Cardiology Division
University of Iowa
IOWA CITY, IA 52242, U.S.A.

Richard I. Kitney, M.D.
Biomedical Systems Group
Dept. of Electrical Engineering
Imperial College, Exhibition Road
LONDON SW5, Great Britain

David Linker M.D.
Regionsykehuset
Inst. for Biomidisinsk Teknikk
Erik Jarls gt 4
N-7006 TRONDHEIM, Norway

Roy W. Martin M.D.
University of Washington
Anaesthesiology/Bioengineering
Main stop RN-10
SEATTLE, WA 98195, U.S.A.

Prof. J. Roelandt, M.D.
University Hospital Rotterdam-Dijkzigt
Thoraxcentre, Bd 408
Dr Molewaterplein 40
NL-3015 GD, ROTTERDAM

H. ten Hoff, M.Sc.
Erasmus University Rotterdam
Thoraxcentre Ee 2302
P.O. Box 1738
NL-3000 DR, ROTTERDAM

Paul G. Yock, M.D.
Cardiac Cath. Lab.
UCSF Dept. of Medicine
Moffit Hospital, Room 1186
SAN FRANCISCO, CA 94143, U.S.A.

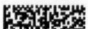